ORTHOPAEDIC SURGERY
OF THE LIMBS IN PARAPLEGIA

BY

L. S. MICHAELIS
M.D. BERLIN, L.R.C.P. AND S. EDINBURGH

WITH 30 ILLUSTRATIONS

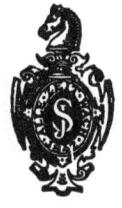

SPRINGER-VERLAG
BERLIN · GÖTTINGEN · HEIDELBERG
1964

From the National Spinal Injuries Centre, Stoke Mandeville Hospital, Bucks/England
(Director: L. Guttmann, C.B.E., M.D., F.R.C.P., F.R.C.S., Hon. D.CH.)

© by Springer-Verlag OHG., Berlin · Göttingen · Heidelberg 1964

Library of Congress Catalog Card Number 64 — 21 007

ISBN 978-3-540-03182-6   ISBN 978-3-642-48242-7 (eBook)
DOI 10.1007/978-3-642-48242-7

Titel-Nr. 1228

Foreword

In the rehabilitation of paraplegics reconstructive and corrective operations play a not unimportant part. Their chief value lies in assisting conservative measures as a means of speeding up the social reintegration of these severely disabled people. Furthermore, in certain groups of paraplegics, these operations establish the very basis for a successful rehabilitation. This applies in the first place to that group of spastic and flaccid paraplegics where inadequate early treatment has led to severe tendon and joint contractures, secondly to that group of paraplegics who develop para-articular ossification of so far unexplained aetiology.

The complex problems we meet in the rehabilitation of paraplegics demand exact indications for reconstructive and corrective operations. To fit them suitably into the overall-plan of treatment demands proper knowledge of the neurophysiology of spinal man.

In almost twenty years a certain system of reconstructive and corrective operations has been developed at the National Spinal Injuries Centre, Stoke Mandeville. Dr. MICHAELIS, who has acquired considerable experience in the techniques of this operative and post-operative treatment, undertook the commendable task of presenting these in a monograph. The special value of this publication lies in the description not only of the successes but also of the failures of operative treatment.

I hope that this monograph will be a valuable help and guide for all doctors, whose responsible task and goal it is to achieve the social reintegration of the paraplegic.

LUDWIG GUTTMANN

Preface

,,The orthopaedic surgery of paraplegics is a virgin field, with no text-book to tell us what to do."

L. F. MILLER (1956)

Although FOERSTER, MUNRO, GUTTMANN, BORS, COMARR, MERLE d'AUBIGNÉ and BÉNASSY, GINGRAS, HARDY and MASSE have reported on experience with major series of operations, particularly for spasticity, there exists, as yet, no survey of a comparatively large and comprehensive material which also includes other operations on the limbs of paraplegics.

A detailed description of the operative and post-operative techniques which have stood the test of time may be welcome.

In 1950 I became an apprentice once more. Dr. GUTTMANN taught me how to adapt an experience of 20 years in orthopaedic surgery to his plan for the rehabilitation of the paraplegic. There was much to learn, since none of the various consequences of a cord injury can be considered or treated in isolation.

Spinal man develops his own physiology which neurology, medicine, urology and general, plastic and orthopaedic surgery have to take into account. Research and nursing, indication and operative technique demand wide knowledge of the interplay between the functions of the paraplegic. Those who intend to treat him will have to be his general doctors first, from whichever specialty they might approach the complex problems of the treatment of injury to the spinal cord.

A large part of my time has since been devoted to the general treatment of our patients.

The theme of this book is the operative orthopaedic work of these 12 years. Even seemingly unimportant detail as for example the average duration of anaesthesia and operation will have to be mentioned. In the treatment of the paraplegic there is no such thing as "unimportant detail".

My thanks are due in the first place to Dr. GUTTMANN who entrusted me with a large part of the operative orthopaedics on his patients and helped me to improve the presentation. My colleague, Dr. JACK WALSH, who as Dr. GUTTMANNS deputy is responsible for the greater part of the surgery of the Centre, has, in earlier years, often assisted me. His help was invaluable. My colleagues, Dr. JOHN SILVER and Dr. J. R. DOGGART, have helped me with constructive criticism of the text. Dr. NORMAN WELPLY, the ideal anaesthetist of the Centre, has kindly contributed a short chapter on Anaesthesia in Paraplegics. To other colleagues, as well as to the sisters, nurses, orderlies and physiotherapists who helped me in looking after my patients, my thanks must go collectively.

L. S. M.

Contents

Introduction:
General surgical technique of operations on the limbs of paraplegics

Several of the operations to be described here use the classical methods of orthopaedic surgery. Some have been modified in details of technique and a few have been devised by the writer to serve purposes peculiar to the pathological conditions met with in paraplegics.

Among the consequences of paraplegia which demand the constant attention of the surgeon, the threat of ischaemia and the loss of sensation particularly endanger the success of operations and of post-operative treatment.

Loss of tissue-tone in the early stages, and atrophy and fibrosis in the later stages of paraplegia combine with the disturbance of vasomotor-control in demanding special precautions which will have to be taken, if pressure sores, haemorrhage and infection are to be prevented. A tourniquet should not be used.

A *high level of haemoglobin* — at least 90% in men, 85% in women — is one of the principal safeguards before, during and after an operation. No operation should be undertaken unless these levels have been reached, if necessary with the aid of preoperative blood-transfusions.

In all operations on patients paralysed at upper dorsal and at cervical levels, and on older people, blood-transfusion should start as soon as the patient is on the operating-table. It should be continued until the patient has been returned to his bed.

Within three days of the operation, the haemoglobin-level should, in all cases, be checked and further transfusion given if needed. (See also under Anaesthesia.)

During operation, *haemostasis* has to be very thorough. Even small vessels bleed more profusely and for a longer period than in the non-paraplegic. The vasomotor-control of paraplegics cannot be relied on, and even small haematomata provide a breeding ground for infective organisms in devitalised tissue.

Haemostasis by coagulation-diathermy has proved the most dependable method. Ligation of vessels should be reduced to a minimum, since the common materials used for ligature and suture (catgut, thread, silk and nylon) act as irritants which are not absorbed or encapsulated as efficiently as in normal tissues. Not rarely they are expelled through stitch fistulae, even years after an operation.

With the exception of occasional ligatures of major vessels and a continuous suture of the peritoneum, stainless steel wire has been used exclusively as our *suture-material*, both for buried and for skin sutures. Gauge 40 is sufficiently strong for most purposes. In certain cases, gauge 36 had to be used. With this wire, the foreign-body reaction was insignificant.

Drainage has been avoided except after the operations on the infected hip-joint and after excision of ectopic bone, where even small accumulations of blood or serum have to be guarded against. Our results show that drainage is not needed in other operations on the paralysed limb.

In order *to prevent infection*, the skin has to be thoroughly prepared with three consecutive applications of mild antiseptic solution — flavine — in the 36 hours preceding the operation. In operations on bones and joints and in tendon-transfer the incision has been made through a sterile stockinet cover. Before closure, the wounds have been sprayed with an antibiotic

Postoperatively the surgeon will have to examine the patient and the dressing every day. Dressings hardened by clotted blood have to be changed since they may cause skin defects through friction. Bladder-function has to be checked, since after operation the well-established automatism may be disturbed.

Drugs should be sparingly used. Analgesics are rarely needed, antispastics rarely effective.

The limb has to be put into the appropriate *position* and maintained in it. *Treatment by passive movement* has to be started and individually devised from the first post-operative day onwards and, in certain cases, carried out by the surgeon himself for the first few weeks.

When *splints* are being employed, they will have to be made, padded, put in position, removed and re-applied by the surgeon himself. In patients with severe spasticity, he will have to remove them daily, inspect the skin, re-pad and adjust the splint. Only thus can pressure-sores be prevented.

Anaesthesia

By

Dr. NORMAN WELPLY
M.B.E., M.R.C.S., L.R.C.P., D.A.

Patients paralysed below T. 6 react to a general anaesthetic like normal people. No special precautions are necessary. Patients with higher dorsal and cervical lesions present certain problems, since —

1. the vasomotor-control is unreliable or absent,
2. the intercostal muscles are incompletely or completely paralysed.

In such cases the following precautions are needed:

a) only small doses of Thiopentone (see page 3).

b) only small doses of relaxants, since otherwise apnoea is prolonged (see page 3). (It is often found that apnoea is prolonged in old cases of poliomyelitis, even when the dose is reduced.)

c) Shock must be foreseen and prevented by appropriate blood-transfusion.

A patient with a cervical lesion may collapse without warning. One moment he reacts normally and the next moment he is deathly pale and sweating and his pulse is fast and thready. There is no gradual decline as in the non-paralysed patient. For this reason, blood-transfusion starts in all major operations as soon as the patient is on the table. An injection of Phenergan (promethazine hydrochloride) 50 mgr. with, or one hour before, the premedication has proved invaluable in the prevention of collapse.

d) All patients are intubated. This makes sure of free gas-exchange and, in experienced hands, has no drawbacks.

a) Details

The main point is sufficient depth during induction for intubation, followed by a very light maintenance.

In those complete lesions, where the main reason for anaesthesia is the suppression of spasticity, these very small doses suffice and no further relaxants are needed.

In incomplete lesions further small amounts of relaxants may become necessary. During obturator neurectomy, too large a dose might mask the effect of electrical stimulation of the nerve. Controlled respiration is not recommended, since it throws additional strain on the heart and increases the danger of collapse.

b) Typical anaesthesia

A. *Lesions below T. 6.*

Premedication: intramuscular injection Omnopon (Pantopon) 20 mgms. Atropin 0.6 mgms. one hour before operation.

Induction: Thiopentone (Pentothal) 500 mgr. and Gallamine (Flaxedil) 80 mgms. followed by intubation.

Maintenance: Nitrous oxide and oxygen with the semi-open circuit with a little Trilene or intravenous injection of Pethilorfan 50 mgms.

B. *High dorsal and cervical lesions.*

Premedication: intramuscular injection Pethilorfan (Lorfalgyl) 50 mgms. Atropin 0.6 mgms. one hour before operation.

Induction: Thiopentone, about 300 mgr., Flaxedil 40—60 mgr. followed by intubation.

Maintenance: Nitrous oxide and oxygen in the semi-open circuit is generally sufficient. Very small quantities of Trilene may occasionally be added.

In this type of light anaesthesia Fluothane has no advantages over Trilene and the great drawback is that it causes restlessness after operation.

If the patient collapses during anaesthesia, this can be corrected by speeding up the transfusion and by small doses of vasopressor drugs. But these must be used with the greatest caution. 4 mgms. of Vasoxine (methoxamine hydrochloride, Vasosteril) may — in high lesions — raise the blood-pressure by 100 mm.

Neurological terminology

In order to prevent misunderstanding, some neurological terms will be defined here as simply as possible. Basic knowledge of the neurology of the spinal cord is taken for granted.

The level of paraplegia is determined and called after the lowest intact neurological segment of the spinal cord, not after the number of a possibly fractured vertebra. For example, a lesion below C 6 causes signs of neurological deficit in the seventh cervical segment and below.

Complete and incomplete paraplegia: Paralysis may be complete. This means that all normal motor and sensory function, together with that of the bladder, the bowels and the sexual organs, is abolished. The higher the complete paraplegia, the greater the disturbance of vasomotor control and temperature-regulation. Or paralysis may be incomplete. This term includes a great variety of combinations of neurological signs, from a slight spastic paresis to the nearly complete transverse syndrome.

Spastic paraplegia: The form of spinal paralysis which follows a transverse lesion of the cord above the conus medullaris. It may be part of a complete or incomplete paraplegia. Spasms are the result of uninhibited reflex activity in the cord which has isolated by injury or disease, and been deprived of the regulating influence of cerebral pathways, in particular the pyramidal tracts.

Flaccid paraplegia: The form of spinal paralysis which follows injury or disease of the lower motor-neuron, as for example in cauda equina lesions or in damage which extends not only transversely but also longitudinally within the cord and affects the anterior horns of the isolated cord (GUTTMANN 1942).

In cervical and conus-lesions, mixed forms of spastic and flaccid paralysis may exist.

Paralysis of autonomic mechanisms accompanies spastic and flaccid paraplegia and affects the function of the bladder, bowels and sex organs. It is also responsible for the extensive changes in the functions of respiration, circulation and sweating.

General statistics

The total number of all patients of the National Spinal Injuries Centre from February 1944 to the 31. August 1962 was *2,857*. In 294 patients (10.1%) orthopaedic operations became necessary. 227 patients were operated on by the writer and 459 operations were carried out.

Among the 227 patients, there were 158 men, 58 women and 11 children.

Table 1		Table 2	
Age groups		*Level of Paraplegia*	
1—13 years	11	Cervical	63
14—20 years	38	T. 1—5	29
21—30 years	76	T. 6—10	68
31—40 years	37	T. 11 and bel.	51
41—50 years	40	Cauda equina.	11
51—60 years	19	Cerebral	2
61—70 years	5	Poliomyelitis	3
over 70 years	1		227
	227		

The great majority of patients who required operations, 186, had spastic lesions. 41 had flaccid lesions. Of these, 159 had incomplete, 68 complete lesions.

Table 3. *Time elapsed between onset of paraplegia and admission to the Centre*

Less than 24 hours	14	(Immediate admissions)
1 day — 3 weeks	17	(Early admissions)
3 weeks — 6 months	30	
6 months — 1 year	36	
1 year — 5 years	64	
6 years — 10 years	34	
11 years — 20 years	25	
More than 20 years	7	
	227	

Only 6 operations on immediate admissions, 7 on early admissions had later to be done for spasticity; the other 18 operations dealt with associated fractures of the long bones.

Table 4. *The cause of paraplegia*

Trauma		*Disease of the spinal cord*		*Disease of the Spine*	
Gunshot wound	14	Transverse myelitis	16	Prolapsed intervertebral disc	6
Bomb	2	Epidural abscess	12	Pott's disease	4
Stab wound	1	Disseminated sclerosis	19	Spondylosis	3
Traffic accidents	62	Tumour of the cord	20	Paget's disease	1
Accidents at work	20	Vascular accident	10	Haemangioma of vertebra	1
Accidents at home	8	Arachnoiditis	4	Sarcoid	1
Sports accidents	14	Spina bifida (myelocele)	4		16
	121	Poliomyelitis	3		
		Cerebral damage	2		
			90		

Total: 227

Disease of the cord or spine accounted for nearly a half of the 227 operation cases, but represents only a third of our total material of 2,857 patients. This difference is explained by the relatively large number of patients with disseminated sclerosis and tumor of the cord who were admitted especially for the operations.

Table 5. *Indications for operations*

For spasticity and contracture	392
Other indications	67

Upper extremity		*Lower extremity*	
Fractures of the long bones	8	Fractures of the long bones	10
Tendon transfers	7	*Hip-joint*	
Para-articular ossification		Sepsis	12
at the elbow	2	Para-articular ossification	9
Arthrodesis of wrist	1	*Knee-joint*	
Meniscus of wrist	1	Ankylosis in extension	7
		Limitation of flexion	2
		Toes	
		Keller's operation	3
		Amputation	5
	19		48 = 67

Total   459 operations

Operations are counted as incisions, but iliopsoas myotomy is counted separately, even if done together with obturator neurectomy. Tendon transfers and multiple subcutaneous tenotomies of toes are counted once only.

For further detail, see special statistics in their chapters.

Table 6. *Anaesthesia*

General   314
Local   2
                   None   17
316 (459 operations)

Quite often more than one operation could be done under the same anaesthetic.

Table 7. *Follow-up*

Re-examined after —

1—6 months	65 patients
7 months—1 year	28 patients
2 years	36 patients
3 years	24 patients
4 years	18 patients
5 years	12 patients
6 years	5 patients
7 years	7 patients
8 years	12 patients
9 years	14 patients
10—12 years	6 patients
	227

A. Operations for spasticity and contracture

In most instances it is possible to reduce spasticity and prevent contractures by proper positioning of the patient from the first day onwards.

Prevention of contractures. In cervical lesions, particularly those below C 6, the arms must be kept extended to prevent flexion contracture at the elbow joint due to shortening of the intact biceps while overstretching of the paralysed triceps should be avoided. The wrist should be held in about 20° extension, with the fingers slightly flexed around a cotton-wool roll.

While on their backs, all patients' hips and knees should lie in full extension, the legs being abducted at the hips with pillows between the knees. When turned on their side, the patients' hips and knees should be flexed.

In all positions, the ankle must be kept at a right angle, not by splints which cause pressure-sores and peroneal palsy, but by firmly supported pillows placed against the soles. If this positioning is not practised and if passive movements through the full range of every joint are not carried out daily and repeatedly, then contracture will supervene. Spasticity, developing in or after the third week after the accident, will start off the vicious circle. Contracture will provide the stimulus for spasticity which, in turn, will increase the degree of contracture (GUTTMANN 1953).

The level of injury or distribution of the disease of the pyramidal tract determines the muscle groups in which spasticity will develop.

The purpose of orthopaedic operations is either to interrupt the reflex arc, and so render a muscle group flaccid, or to reduce the excitability of the cord by correcting the contractures. HARDY (1959) calls these operations ,,destructive", because they involve division of nerves, muscle or tendons. This is hardly justified. Anatomical elimination is only the basis for constructive restoration of one or more functions).

The right time for an operation. Before deciding on the *right time for an operation*, four sets of questions have to be answered:

1. Have all factors been removed which are known to increase spasticity?
   In particular, is there severe infection or distension in the urinary tract?
   Are there stones, orchitis, phimosis?
   Is the patient constipated?
   Are there haemorrhoids, an active gastric or duodenal ulcer?
   Are there pressure sores?
   Is he anaemic?
   Is there a paronychia?
2. Have all conservative means been tried and found wanting?
3. Does operation hold out the promise of correction of deformity and reduction of spasticity beyond its local effect?
4. Is there a danger of harmful consequences, e.g., may antagonistic muscle-groups be given a chance of producing new contractures (abduction at the hip, genu recurvatum at the knee)?

The right type of operation has to be chosen just as carefully as the time. Often there is no doubt about it. When, in attempts at standing, a spastic pes equinus is predominant in a violent flexion-synergy, elongation of the Achilles-tendon may be sufficient as the only operative procedure.

When flexion-contracture at the knee prevents the wearing of calipers or recovery of the quadriceps, tenomyotomy of the superficial knee-flexors may help.

In severe adduction-spasm or-contracture of the hip, obturator neurectomy might be indicated, in flexion-contracture of the hip iliopsoas myotomy.

Multiple operations. Often several of these contractures exist together and, in most cases, they are bilateral. There remains the question of where to start and whether on both sides at once or unilaterally to begin with. Only experience and possibly the existence of a clear trigger-point can give the answer.

Spasticity may diminish over the whole leg after correction of only one deformity; in some cases, even of the other leg as well. (GUTTMANN 1954, ABRAMSON 1962).

Proper choice of the right type of operation at the right time may save the patient several operations. But the surgeon may be disappointed and a new operation may have to be done under another anaesthetic which one could have included under the first. In some cases one may suspect at the first operation, that, more likely than not, further operations will have to be done. But it is better to give the patient the chance of achieving the desired result with a minimum of surgery, before deciding upon further measures.

The intrathecal alcohol block. Finally, there are patients with the most severe triple contractures at hip, knee and ankle, where one has to consider the radical solution, the *intrathecal alcohol block*. This method may have to be employed also in cases where several peripheral operations were unsuccessful.

The intrathecal alcohol block was introduced by DOGLIOTTI (1931) for the treatment of intractable pain in carcinomatosis, but given up because it produced paralysis in normal patients. It was first used by GUTTMANN (1946) for the treatment of intractable spasticity in complete paraplegia.

BORS (1948) and GINGRAS (1948) injected 8—15 ml. of absolute alcohol into the subarachnoid space. This method has proved very effective in Guttmann's hands, although he never injects more than 10 ml. It has to be reserved for selected cases and must be carried out carefully. It is particularly useful for the treatment of intractable spasticity in complete lesions. In some cases, especially in cervical lesions, the alcohol block may have to be used in incomplete lesions also, although this means that an automatic bladder will become flaccid and that sexual function is lost.

The intrathecal injection of phenol in glycerin was first recommended by MAHER (1955), again for the treatment of severe pain in carcinomatosis. NATHAN (1958, 1959), BROWN (1958) and KELLY and GAUTHIER-SMITH (1959) used selective injections of phenol with the intention of abolishing spasticity only without disturbing the function of a normal bladder. With this method abolition of spasticity appears to be less reliable than with the alcohol block and prolonged disturbance of bladder function can not be avoided with any certainty.

Operations for spasticity and contracture: general statistics

Table 8. *Operations — 392*

Operation	No. of operations
Obturator neurectomy	102
Iliopsoas myotomy	15
Tenomyotomy of knee flexors	108
Elongation of tendo Achilles	129
Tenotomy of posterior tibial tendon	3
Tendon-transfer for —	
Pes equinovarus	3
Pes equinovalgus	1
Neurotomy of peroneal nerve	2
Toes:	
Subcutaneous tenotomies etc.	19
Hip:	
For limitation of extension, flaccid	5
For subluxation combined with	
adduction- and flexion-contracture	1
Knee:	
For flexion contracture, spastic	1
For flexion contracture, flaccid	2
For extension contracture, flaccid	1
Total Operations:	392

Table 9. *Number of operations per patient*

1 operation	60 patients	60 operations
2 operations	62 patients	124 operations
3 operations	23 patients	69 operations
4 operations	18 patients	72 operations
5 and more operations	10 patients	67 operations
	173 patients	392 operations

Common operations
1. Obturator neurectomy for spastic adduction contracture at the hip

(after SELIG, 1914)

Table 10. *Statistics: Neurological Symptomatology*

Level	Complete	Incomplete
Cervical	—	31*
T. 1—5	2	7
T. 6—10	11	19
T. 11 and below	1	7
	14	64 = 78 patients

* Patients with disseminated sclerosis are counted as incomplete cervical lesions.

Table 11

Operation on one side only in 46 patients	Obturator neurectomy alone in 28 patients
on both sides in 32 patients	*Combined with:*
(of these simultaneous in 18 patients)	Iliopsoas myotomy in 8 patients
78 patients	Tenomyotomy of knee-flexors in 22 patients
	Elongation of Achilles tendon in 14 patients
	Other operations 6 patients
	78 patients

a) Technique of the operation

Positioning: On a thick sponge-rubber mattress the patient lies either flat on his back or slightly turned towards the operator, a pillow supporting the opposite side of the pelvis.

Towelling: The abdominal wall and, below the groin, the inside of the thigh are exposed, surrounded by towelling fixed at the umbilicus, symphysis, iliac spine and a point 4″ distal to the centre of the inguinal ligament. The diathermy electrode is fixed to the opposite thigh.

Incision and procedure: An oblique 8″ straight incision is made from a point 1″ medial to the iliac spine to a point 1″ proximal and lateral to the symphysis pubis. Exact haemostasis. The aponeurosis of external oblique is split in the same direction and length as the skin incision. At a right angle to and from the centre of this incision laterally, the fasciae propriae of the internal oblique and transversus muscles are divided.

Between their muscle-bundles the tips of the forefingers gently move deeper, pushing medially the peritoneum and extraperitoneal fat. The pulse of the external iliac artery is easily felt. The fingers proceed on its medial aspect where the larger vein can be seen and felt. If there is only a small amount of loose extraperitoneal fat and the muscles are weak, a long and wide retractor can be introduced at the proximal corner and medially. It is gently eased into the depth of the cavity. In some cases, it is necessary to split the internal oblique and transversus muscles for an inch or so parallel to the skin incision. Haemostasis.

In simple cases it is now possible to feel rather than see the nerve, deep to the vein and running parallel with it. It is 4—5 mm. thick, hard and taut. More often, fat and adhesions have to be pushed gently off it with small swabs in long forceps.

Working gently saves time, since all bleeding is avoided. In difficult cases, after chronic inflammation in the pelvis, the nerve may be invisible and impossible to feel and has to be isolated from massive dense fibrous adhesions. Once more patience is rewarded by a saving of time, since bleeding at this depth demands tedious haemostasis. Once the nerve is free for about 2", two Kocher forceps are applied to it, as high as convenient and at about 1" distance from each other. Contraction

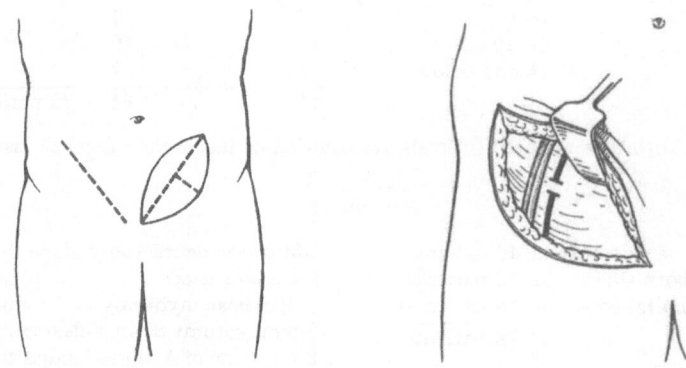

Fig. 1   Fig. 2

Fig. 1. Obturator-Neurectomy 1. On right: skin incision. On left: incision of aponeurosis of obl. ext. incision of transv. and obl. int.

Fig. 2. Obturator-Neurectomy 2. On right side. Retractor covers peritoneum. Nerve excised proximally, deep to A. und V. iliaca ext.

of the adductors can be seen in the field left free on the thigh and is proof that the nerve was properly identified.

If in doubt, one can touch the nerve with the diathermy electrode under reduced current (but see Anaesthesia p. 3). If there is no definite contraction of the adductors, one has to make sure that the ductus deferens, the round ligament or even the ureter have not been mistaken for the nerve. They are much softer and less taut than the nerve, but may run close to and parallel with it.

Once identification is certain, a half-inch piece of the nerve between the forceps is excised. It may be sent for histological examination. It is best to tie the nerve-ends with fine thread, since small vessels here may bleed embarrassingly.

After removal of the forceps the extraperitoneal space is carefully searched for bleeding points which are all coagulated with diathermy. Antibiotic powder is blown in, the retractor removed and muscle, fascia, subcutaneous tissue and skin are sutured with interrupted stitches, constant watch being kept for bleeding points. Where the muscle is strong and very spastic, wire gauge 36 may be used. Otherwise gauge 40 is sufficient for all layers. Where subcutaneous fat is not abundant, no subcutaneous sutures are needed.

Dressing: After the skin has been cleared of blood-spots, it is painted with flavine in spirit and dressed with gauze. This is covered and sealed off with elastoplast.

The patient is carefully lifted on to the trolley and, when he is put into bed, he is turned on his side. Two or more pillows are placed between the knees. This is now easy to do, even after only one-sided neurectomy. Three-hourly-turns, on the back and both sides, can be continued.

As soon as the patient has recovered from the anaesthetic, he should be encouraged to drink small quantities of water at short intervals. Where no stay-catheter is employed, emptying of the bladder must be made sure of and, at times, catheterisation is needed the same evening.

Simultaneous bilateral operation is done from two corresponding incisions on either side. The long transverse or medial longitudinal incisions are not used, since they cross the bladder-region and may interfere with voiding.

Tenotomy of the adductor-tendon is quite superfluous, since, after neurectomy, passive stretching of the now flaccid adductors is easily achieved within a week. COMARR (1960) uses an incision in the medial groin and divides the muscle or tendon of all adductors as well as the branches of the obturator nerve. I prefer to avoid incisions and scars in the skin of the groin, where perspiration may interfere with healing.

Obturator neurectomy may be very easy but, at times, is quite difficult. The operation normally takes about 20 minutes but, in rare cases, may last up to an hour.

b) Postoperative treatment

The dressing should be checked by the surgeon on the first day and changed if it is hardened by clotted blood.

Passive movements start on the first day and consist of gentle abduction at the hip. If this is done too enthusiastically, tears appear in the muscle, accompanied by haemorrhage and swelling, which enforce rest and produce fibrotic scars. A true angle of abduction of 30° is sufficient. During these exercises, a second physio-therapist has to fix the other leg and with it the pelvis.

Stitches are removed by the surgeon on the 10th day and a protective dressing is applied for another few days. In the afternoon, the patient may sit up in the wheelchair. Next morning, he can begin standing and walking exercises, if he had been doing these before the operation.

The final result of the operation, particularly its remote influence on spasticity in the operated limb and the other leg, cannot, in general, be assessed for two to three weeks.

c) Complications and mistakes

Haemorrhage: In one case, the edge of the retractor tore the circumflex iliac vein from the external iliac vein, which had to be tied. The operation had to be abandoned. In another case, an unusually strong inferior epigastric vein was cut while extending the incision through the aponeurosis of the external oblique. Blood flooded the field of operation. Haemostasis took 10 minutes.

Tears in the peritoneum: In three cases, the peritoneum tore during blunt removal of extraperitoneal adhesions. Immediate closure with a fine continuous catgut suture was carried out.

Infection due to missed swab: On one occasion, a small gauze swab was discharged from an abscess 4 weeks after operation. Healing was not further disturbed.

Incomplete neurectomy: In the first year I twice divided only the superficial branch of the nerve, because the neurectomy was done too far distally.

The nerve divides high, or an accessory nerve is present, in about a quarter of all patients (29% according to Gray's Anatomy). Since we always do a high excision, we have had no failure.

Table 12. *Obturator Neurectomy. Results*

Patients 78	Operations 102
Desired local effect	99
Expected distant effect	93
Unexpected distant effect	3
Insufficient effect within the total plan.	9
Complications and mistakes	8

The desired local effect is the correction of adduction-contracture and reduction of spasticity at the hip. The expected distant effect consists of reduction of spasticity elsewhere. Coitus may be rendered possible but, at times, erections and control of an automatic bladder are temporarily weakened.

The unexpected distant effect was the appearance of abduction contracture at the hip. Too drastic abduction and overstretching of the flaccid adductors permitted the spastic gluteus medius to fix the leg almost permanently in abduction.

Summary

Obturator neurectomy — without adductor tenotomy — has proved to be an effective and reliable procedure for the abolition of adductor spasticity and adduction-contracture at the hip. Following this operation continuous maintenance of abduction and immediate passive abduction exercises succed in achieving a satisfactory permanent result.

2. Iliopsoas myotomy for spastic flexion-contracture at the hip

Table 13. *Neurological Symptomatology*

Level	Complete	Incomplete	Operations
Cervical	—	2	4
T. 1—5	—	2	3
T. 6—10	—	3	6
T. 11 and below	—	1	2
Patients		8	15 Operations

Iliopsoas myotomy was added to obturator neurectomy, when spastic flexion-contracture accompanied adduction-contracture. It was done on one side only in one patient and bilaterally in 7 patients; in one patient, the bilateral operation was carried out under one anaesthetic.

Severe spastic flexion contracture at the hip is one of the most serious disabilities for the patient. Standing is made impossible and attempts to correct the deformity by physiotherapy only result in increased lordosis.

Spasticity never relaxes and interferes with sleep. If combined with adduction-contracture, it renders catheterising the patient, or keeping him clean, virtually impossible.

Both deformities can be removed, or at least much reduced, by alcohol block in complete lesions. In incomplete lesions, this radical method should be used in extreme cases only; in particular, where bladder-function is already impaired.

Until a few years ago, results of operations at the distal end of iliopsoas were unsatisfactory, since they corrected only a minor part of the shortening and did nothing to stop spasticity. I decided to divide the muscle-belly proximally on the ilium. The proximal part could then retract while the distal part would be denervated and flaccid and could be stretched.

Division of iliopsoas and rectus abdominis together from a large transverse incision had already been done by FOWLER (1957), in cases of severe disseminated sclerosis. For such cases, we prefer the intrathecal alcohol block. Our method is meant to serve patients with incomplete lesions who, with its help, can be made to stand and walk. Further, we avoid the long transverse incision because it crosses the region of the bladder (see p. 11).

a) Technique of the operation

Positioning: As for obturator neurectomy (p. 9).

Towelling: Towelling is applied as for obturator neurectomy, except that the legs are towelled off separately. Even after anaesthesia has suppressed spasticity, they are still strongly flexed and have to be supported by pillows until, after division of the muscle, they can be extended.

Incision and procedure. As for obturator neurectomy. In cases in which both operations are being combined, the neurectomy should be done first. Then the lateral edge of the skin is retracted laterally. The iliac fascia is split lengthwise. The femoral nerve is gently freed and held aside with a soft sling.

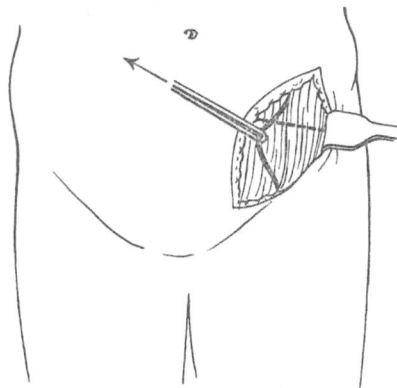

Fig. 3. Iliopsoas Myotomy 1. On left side. Skin retracted laterally. N. femoralis retracted medially with soft sling. Site of transverse division of mm. psoas and iliacus

A long, narrow ringhandle-spike is now inserted between the iliacus muscle and the periosteum of the iliac bone. As far proximally as can be done without undue pulling, two Kocher forceps are clamped on suitable sections of the psoas, which is divided between them with the diathermy knife. This procedure is continued step by step, coagulating the muscle surfaces at each stage. After some 4 or 5 such steps, the iliacus muscle lies exposed and has to be divided completely across. The closer the diathermy knife approaches the deepest and most medial border of the ilium, the closer it approaches the iliac artery.

Now a strip of bone-surface is visible from one border of the ilium to the other. The proximal, spastic parts of the muscle-bellies retract proximally.

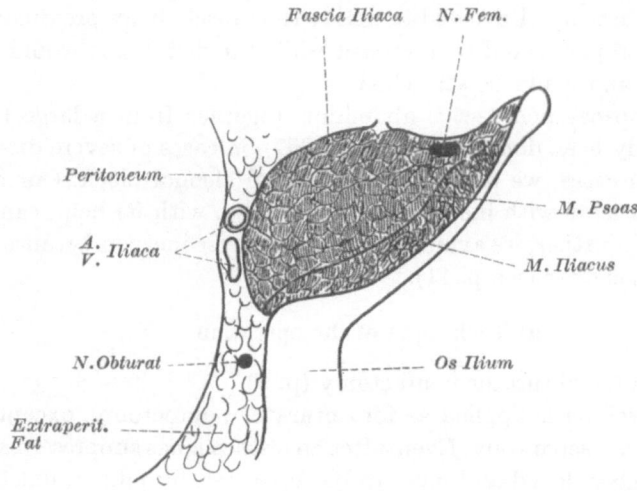

Fig. 4. Iliopsoas Myotomy 2

The surgeon now presses the knee slowly but strongly downwards. He can follow the gliding movement of the distal section and see an ever wider band of ilium. A 1″—2″ gap is needed until the hip is extended and the shortening corrected.

After further haemostasis antibiotic is blown in, the femoral nerve released, and fascia and skin are closed with interrupted wire (gauge 40) sutures.

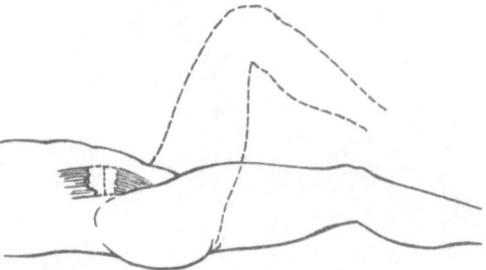

Fig. 5. Iliopsoas Myotomy 3. Lateral view. After complete division of muscles the leg can be extended.
Note: wide muscle-gap

Dressing: As for obturator neurectomy.

b) Postoperative treatment

This differs in some respects from that after neurectomy. The leg is positioned in bed as extended as possible and in slight abduction. During the first 2 weeks only abduction exercises are done. Again stitches are removed on the 10th day, but the patient does not get up before the third week, and then spends increasing periods in his wheelchair. If there has been no sign whatever of deep bleeding, he can start standing exercises after three weeks and, later on, have passive extension-exercises, should that be necessary.

c) Complications and mistakes

Early bleeding: In a woman of 60 with a cervical lesion, we had to re-open the incision on the evening of the day of operation, since it was impossible to be sure from where the bleeding came. The cut surfaces of the muscle were dry. Bleeding originated in several small vessels in the very lax subcutaneous tissue and was easily stopped. Insufficient care in haemostasis was responsible. The final result was not delayed; full extension was achieved and the patient enabled to stand.

Delayed bleeding: In our second patient, we permitted standing exercises after 10 days. This produced a hard swelling under the operation scar without any signs of infection. Absorption of this deep haematoma required three weeks of rest in bed. The final result was not spoilt. A check 3 years later showed an excellent result; the hips in full extension and the patient walking "all day" with elbow crutches.

Table 14. *Iliopsoas Myotomy. Results*

Patients 8	*Operations 15*
Desired local effect	15
Expected distant effect	15
Unexpected distant effect	—
Insufficient effect in general plan	—
Complications and mistakes	2

The desired local effect is the removal of the spastic contracture and the restoration of extension at the hipjoint.

The expected distant effect is the reduction of spasticity in the remainder of the leg and the ability to stand upright.

Summary

Iliopsoas myotomy as described here has proved to be an effective and reliable operation for the reduction of flexion contracture and spasticity at the hip. Late results, in some cases 3 years after the operation, are now available and are in all cases satisfactory.

3. Tenomytomy of the superficial flexors of the knee for spastic flexion contracture

Table 15. *Neurological symptomatology*

Patients: 47 *Level*	*Complete*	*Incomplete*
Cervical	—	23
T. 1—5	2	3
T. 6—10	3	9
T. 11 and below	3	4
	8	39

Table 16

Operations: 108

One sided: 10
Bilateral: 98, of these done at the same time:

inner hamstrings	48 operations	24 patients
both inner, one outer flexor	12 operations	4 patients
both inner and outer flexors	36 operations	9 patients
Repeated	2 operations	
	98 operations	37 patients

Spastic flexion contracture at the knee-joint is a more awkward surgical problem than is usually admitted.

Operation on mild cases may be superfluous because similarly good results can be achieved by physiotherapy alone.

The design of more complicated operations suggests that their authors were dissatisfied with their results.

I have operated on severe contractures only; that is, in cases where extension was limited by 50 to 100 degrees. In several of them, flexion contracture at the knee was secondary to that at the hip.

In the last ten years we have abandoned subcutaneous tenotomy altogether — except at the toes — and rely on an open tenomyotomy.

Before deciding on the operation, we have to consider how great the chances of success will be in cases where there exists also a flexion contracture of the hip-joint. In several cases, deformity at the knee improved greatly after first correcting the contracture at the hip.

a) Technique of the operation

Positioning. Whenever possible, the patient should lie prone. His knees will still be flexed even under the anaesthetic, and the legs will have to be supported by pillows which, after division of muscles and tendons, will have to be removed. Only thus can the result be checked and further division decided on, if necessary.

If there is also considerable flexion contracture at the hip, further pillows will have to support the patient under the abdomen. Great care is needed to prevent pressure on the knee-caps.

In cervical lesions, the prone position may prevent proper ventilation. The patient will then have to be placed on his side and turned when operation is to begin on the second leg.

The majority of patients had simultaneous bilateral division of the inner hamstrings. In some patients, division of the biceps femoris was carried out at the same time.

Towelling. The legs are towelled off separately, leaving free the lower half of the back of the thigh and the flexor-crease of the knee.

Incisions and procedure. These are slightly curved and extend for about 5″ longitudinally through the skin and subcutaneous tissue. They should not reach the flexor crease because of the danger of keloid formation.

After thorough haemostasis, the gracilis and the often very strong bellies of semimembranosus and semitendinosus, with their fasciae propriae, are dissected. They are individually divided with the diathermy knife between Kocher forceps.

After removal of the forceps, the stumps are coagulated. If the proximal ends do not now retract proximally (because of adhesions between them and the superficial fascia or the subcutaneous fat) they have to be freed by blunt dissection with small swabs on long holders. While working with forceps and diathermy for haemostasis, care is needed to avoid damage to the tibial and peroneal nerves which can easily be caught or burned. This may not matter much in complete lesions and may even help to reduce spasticity further. COMARR (1960) recommends neurotomy in some cases.

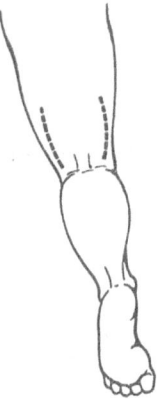

If the tendon of the biceps femoris is to be divided at the same session, this can be done from a corresponding lateral incision.

After an orderly has removed the pillow(s) supporting the legs, the surgeon attempts full extension. If extension cannot be achieved, the structures preventing it will become obvious.

Further division may be necessary and possible, adhesions may have to be divided proximally or the superficial fascia may need transverse division.

Fig. 6.
Tenomyotomy of superficial knee-flexors 1. Medial and lateral skin-incisions. Note: they do not reach flexor crease

After very careful haemostasis, application of antibiotic powder and, where needed, a few subcutaneous wire sutures (gauge 40), the skin is sutured and particularly well adapted. A gauze dressing is applied and is held in position with elastoplast which is fixed with the knee in maximal extension. A wool-mantle is wrapped around the knee and held with an elastic bandage, again with the knee in full extension.

b) Postoperative treatment

In the first 24 hours, the circulation of feet and toes needs watching. The bandage may have to be taken off and re-applied less tightly. The dressing has to be felt for hardening by clotted blood and must be changed if necessary.

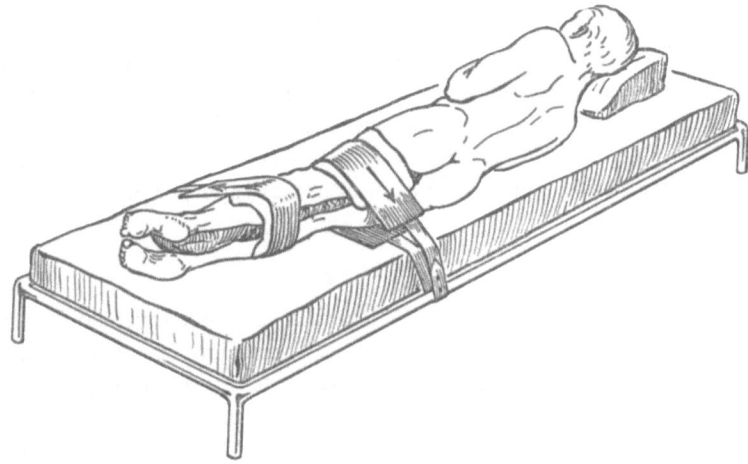

Fig. 7. After Tenomyotomy 2. Legs strapped into extension. Note: pillows between legs and under straps

Maximal extension of the limbs must be maintained throughout. Splints are far too risky and should not be used. Broad canvas straps over thighs and legs, protected by pillows, are tightened at the edge of the bed, pulling in all positions the legs into full extension (GUTTMANN). These straps are only removed and re-applied when the patient is being turned or treated with active and passive movements carried out by the physiotherapist.

These movements start on the first postoperative day. Skin-sutures are removed by the surgeon on the 10th day and a protective dressing is applied for another three days. The patient gets up into the wheelchair and starts walking on the 11th day.

c) Complications and mistakes

1. In one case, the peroneal nerve was permanently damaged, probably by haemostasis proximal to the limit of the incision.

2. *Haemorrhage:* In one case there was delayed bleeding from the proximal muscle-stumps which postponed healing for three weeks. The causes were insufficient haemostasis and, possibly, too enthusiastic passive movements.

3. *Infection:* Infection occurred in this haematoma.

4. *Death:* Two weeks after operation, death occurred in a 62-year-old woman with advanced disseminated sclerosis and hypertension. Four days after operation, she suffered the first stroke, followed ten days later by a second, to which she succumbed.

Table 17. *Tenomyotomy of knee-flexors. Results*

Patients: 47	*Operations:*	*108*
	(subcutaneous:	12)
Desired local effect (occasionally partial)		96
Expected distant effect		96
Unexpected distant effect		—
Insufficient effect in general plan		9
Complications and mistakes		3
Death		1

The desired local effect is correction of the flexion contracture and reduction of spasticity. This was achieved in all cases, at least in part. Only in subcutaneous operations were results unsatisfactory and, in two of them, open operation was performed later. The expected distant effect was reduction of spasticity in the whole leg; this was often achieved but was not always permanent.

Summary

Open tenomyotomy of the superficial flexors of the knee joint can be an effective operation for the reduction of spasticity and correction of contracture. Success depends throughout on proper indication and timing, particularly in relation to a coexisting flexion contracture of the hip, on a careful technique and intensive post-operative treatment (see also Cases I and II, p. 24—26).

4. Elongation of the Achilles tendon for spastic pes equinus

Table 18. *Neurological symptomatology*

Level	Complete	Incomplete
Cervical	—	13
T. 1—5	6	4
T. 6—10	7	25
T. 11 and below	6	13
Cauda equina	1	2
Poliomyelitis		1
Cerebral		1
	20	59
	Patients:	79

Table 19. *Operations*

One-sided only	29	of these simultaneous:	
Bilateral (50 patients)	100	(41 patients)	82
	129 Operations		

a) Technique of the operation

This well-known operation is one which, with proper indication and when done at the right time, will give reliable results. In many cases, the result exceeds correction of deformity and reduces not only the spasticity of the whole leg but also, quite often, the spasticity of the other leg on which no operation was done.

The author has modified the incision and tendon-suture in order to prevent complications even in the most severely spastic patients so that sutures will be safe under the very heavy strain of spastic muscle-contractions immediately after the operation. Tenotomy alone weakens the stability of the ankle. We have used it once only, in a child with cerebral palsy.

Positioning. The patient lies prone. His legs are made to overhang the lower end of the table by about 10″, so that ankle and foot are free.

Towelling. The legs are towelled off separately down to the middle of the calf. Small toe-towels cover the forefoot and toes.

Incision and procedure. This must be long enough to permit proper elongation, so that 2—3″ of the tendon-halves will be available for suture. 10″ is the usual length.

In contrast to operations on non-paralysed patients, the incision lies *lateral* to the tendon, about ¾″, so as to avoid pressure or scraping by the other spastic limb. It should not extend distally to the edge of a shoe, which might later damage the scar by rubbing.

The short saphenous vein may be damaged by the skin incision and, in that case, has to be tied with fine thread. Its transverse branches, particularly at the distal end of the incision, need careful coagulation.

The tendon is exposed by gently pulling the medial skin-edge medially. The paratenon is often thickened and is, at times, fibrous. All layers, even the finest, have to be dissected off the tendon.

Muscle-fibres which, in front of the tendon, often reach to its insertion, should be removed by blunt dissection where possible, but one may leave a thin layer

2*

on the tendon. It will prove a help in the early stages of scar-formation. The Z
division of the tendon should be too long rather than too short, particularly in
cases in which, even under anaesthesia, the angle of the ankle is still about 110
degrees. The longitudinal cut must be exactly in the midline to ensure that both
halves of the sutured tendon are of equal strength. Often it is possible, at this
stage, to achieve sufficient dorsiflexion. Since
the loss of muscle-tone in the gastrocnemius
under anaesthesia has to be considered, an
angle of 85 degrees is needed; 90 degrees is
not enough.

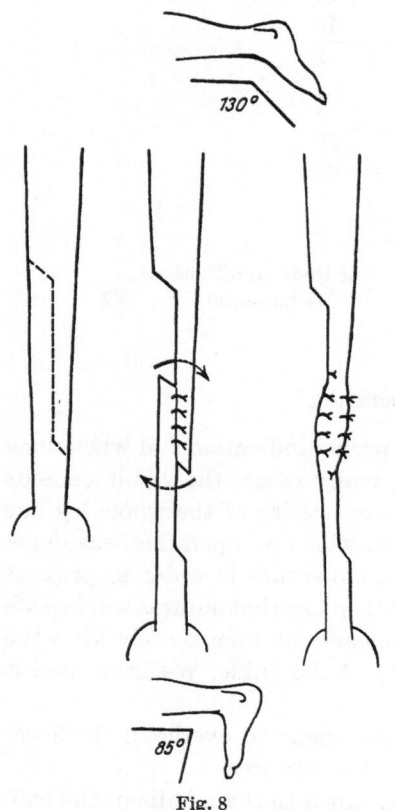

At times, it is necessary to divide the
narrow tendon of the plantaris muscle separately. In a few cases, the fasciae and posterior
capsule of the ankle-joint need division before
the necessary angle can be reached. In such
cases very thorough haemostasis, at the
distal end, is essential.

The suture of the tendon can start now.
The first suture determines the extent of
elongation. It can, therefore, only be inserted
when an angle of 85 degrees has been achieved
and is being held.

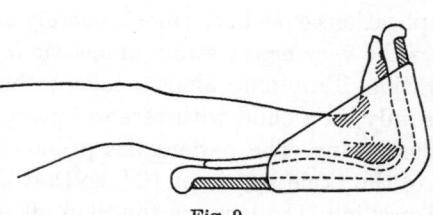

Fig. 8   Fig. 9

Fig. 8. Elongation of Achilles-Tendon. Z-incision, first suture line, second suture line, forming a tube

Fig. 9. Plaster leg-splint, for postoperative treatment after elongation of Achilles-tendon. Note: Thick
padding, 85° angle, maintained by padded diagonal plaster-strips. Splint ends well distal to flexor-
crease of knee. main danger areas for pressure sores: ▨

4 stainless steel wire sutures (gauge 40) unite the adjoining edges, at about
$^1/_3''$ intervals.

The half-united tendon slips are now folded on to each other and their remaining free edges are joined similarly. The proximal and distal ends are adapted by a
further oblique suture each. This double-suture not only is stronger than others,
but also utilises remnants of muscle, now enclosed within a tube of tendon, for
early scar-formation, and provides smooth gliding surfaces around the new tendon.

After thorough haemostasis, the new tendon is replaced in its bed and, after
blowing in powder, the skin is closed with very accurate adaptation.

The gauze dressing is kept in place by elastoplast applied with the ankle
fully corrected. A window must be left over the heel so that redness or blistering
can be discovered immediately.

In bilateral operations, the second tendon is lengthened in the same manner before the special plaster-splints are made and applied.

One-sided operation, including the plaster-splint, takes 45 minutes, while bilateral operation takes 1 ½ hours.

b) Postoperative treatment

The circulation of the toes on the first day has to be controlled and the splint removed. The dressing may have to be changed. Control of the skin of the heel and, when needed, re-padding of the splint, are particularly important. This has to be repeated every other day and, where spasticity is violent, even daily.

On every occasion one has to make sure that the heel really fits closely on to the padded plaster-heel and sole, so that the chosen angle is being preserved. Passive movements of hips, knees and toes continue. On the 10th day, stitches are removed and a protective dressing applied. From now on, the splint is removed once daily by the physiotherapist for passive or, where possible, active movements of the ankle. In a number of such cases, I found after this operation that, after correction of the fixed deformity, the tibialis anticus or extensor digitorum muscles were able to function again; this saved the patient a foot-drop-device and improved his gait.

This second period takes another 10 days. Three weeks after the operation the patient starts standing and walking again. This is particularly important since nothing maintains correction at the ankle as well as weightbearing on the full sole.

c) Complications and mistakes

Pressure-sores under splint. Early redness was discovered at some control-inspections. Repadding caused it to disappear.

Relapses: In two patients, elongation had to be repeated because deformity recurred. The first patient was a 10-year-old girl, in whom I did not allow for rapid growth. The second patient was a 35-year-old man. Passive movements in bed were not carried out energetically enough and the ankle stiffened at about 110 degrees. This second operation proved relatively easy and led to a good and lasting result.

Table 20. *Elongation of the achilles tendon. Results*

Patients: 79	Operations: 129
Desired local effect	127
Expected distant effect	127
Insufficient effect in general plan	—
Complications and mistakes	2

The desired local effect consists once more of correction of deformity and reduction of spasticity. The expected distant effect is all-round improvement of spasticity in the operated leg and, at times, in the opposite leg.

Summary

Elongation of the Achilles tendon for spastic pes equinus is an effective and reliable operation which, given the correct indication, helps to reduce spasticity of the entire limb. With the suture technique as described here, with careful prevention of pressure sores threatened by the plaster-splint, and correct timing of active and passive exercises, no failure was seen.

Rare operations
5. Open tenotomy of the tibialis posterior tendon

In three patients, in whom the varus element in pes equinovarus was very pronounced, we combined tenotomy of tibialis posterior with elongation of the Achilles tendon from a short incision behind the inner malleolus. The results were always satisfactory.

6. Tendon-transfer at the ankle

Occasionally, one sees considerable spastic contracture in conus-lesions which interferes with standing and walking. In three patients we had to operate.

a) Bilateral severely spastic pes equinovarus

A man, aged 39, had a complete conus-lesion below L. 4 after a war injury (gunshot-wound). Spasticity, even after elongation of the Achilles tendon, remained so severe that both feet were forced into extreme varus.

Operative technique (Figs. 10/11). The tibialis anticus tendon was severed at its insertion. From a second, longitudinal, incision over the lower half of the leg, this tendon was pulled up proximally. The tendon of the paralysed extensor digitorum communis was isolated from the same incision and divided just below the muscle-belly.

Foot and toes were brought into dorsiflexion and midposition, not into valgus. The shortened tibialis anticus tendon was then united with the proximal end of the distal part of the extensor digitorum communis tendon. Several wire sutures (gauge 40) were used. After careful haemostasis and closure of both incisions, a thickly padded backsplint of plaster was bandaged on. This was removed daily at first and, later, on alternate days, being repadded when necessary. Skin-sutures were removed after 10 days and the splint was taken off after three weeks. Operation on the other foot followed a fortnight after the first. Two months after the first operation, the patient began to walk. Correction was perfect and spasticity much reduced. The power in the reconstructed extensor digitorum communis balanced the pull of the elongated Achilles tendon. Three years later, the result had been fully maintained.

Fig. 10a u. b. Tendon-Transfers at ankle, first method. a) Skin-incisions. b) Deformity corrected. Tendon of Tib ant. sutured to tendon of ext. dig.

b) Unilateral severely spastic pes equinovarus

With two other patients, another technique (after BIESALSKI and MAYER, 1916) proved so effective that it is described in detail.

Transfer of the tibialis anticus tendon into the sheath of the extensor digitorum communis served both to reduce spasticity and to correct the varus deformity.

1. From a short transverse incision, the tibialis anticus tendon was divided near its insertion.

2. From a 3″ longitudinal incision over the lower half of the leg, the tendons of tibialis anticus and extensor digitorum were exposed.

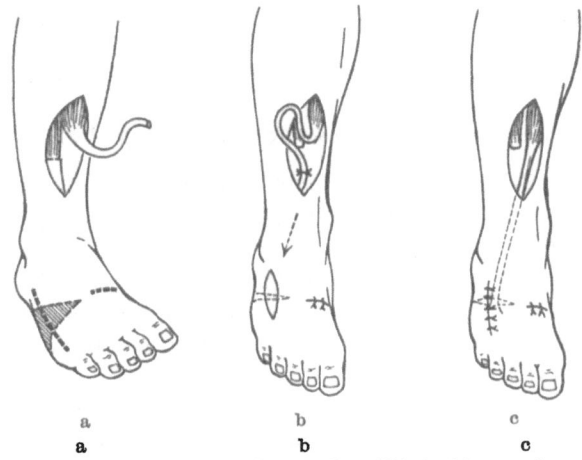

a   b   c

Fig. 11a—c. Tendon-Transfers at ankle, second method. a) Skin incisions and area of resection of bone. b) Tendon of Tib. ant pulled out proximally, temporarily sutured to tendon of ext. dig. P. varus and adduction of forefoot corrected by closing wedge-shaped bone-gap. c) Tendon of ext. dig. pulled down distally and removed. Tendon of tib. ant. now running in its new sheath, fixed to distal edge of bone-gap

3. The tendon of tibialis anticus was pulled out of its sheath from the proximal incision.

4. The tendon of extensor communis was divided at the musculotendineous junction.

5. The distal end of the tibialis anticus tendon was temporarily firmly united with the proximal end of the tendon of extensor digitorum communis.

6. On the dorsum of the foot, the tendons of extensor digitorum communis were exposed through a separate incision.

7. From here, they were drawn out and with them the tendon of tibialis anterior which now lay in the tendon-sheath of extensor digitorum communis.

8. The tendon of extensor digitorum communis was removed. The distal end of the tendon of tibialis anterior was firmly sutured sub-periosteally on the dorsum pedis, with the foot in mid-position, not valgus, and slight dorsiflexion.

9. After thorough haemostasis, all incisions were carefully sutured.

10. A light well-padded plaster-splint held the corrected position at leg and foot.

In one patient, additional correction of the adduction-deformity of the forefoot was achieved through a wide bone wedge-excision from the lateral border.

Union occured in ten weeks. Gait and standing were now all but normal. The patient, who had been self-conscious about his "clubfoot", felt much reassured.

c) Spastic pes equino-valgus

A girl, aged 20, suffered from an incomplete lesion below T. 9 after a motor-cycle accident. Paralysis was complete below L. 4 with severe spastic pes valgus on one side. She just managed to walk with sticks.

Here, the same technique was used, but the peroneal tendons were transferred into the sheath of extensor digitorum communis. Here too, the result was very satisfactory and has remained so for six years.

7. Neurotomy of the peroneal nerve

In two patients the peroneal nerve was exposed behind the head of the fibula and divided. Previous attempts at paralysing it by injection had failed.

8. Subcutaneous tenotomies and corrections of spastic toes

In 19 patients, insufficient early treatment had produced flexion-contractures and hammer toes which, in addition, were severely spastic. Shoes could not be worn since they produced pressure sores.

In 11 cases, subcutaneous tenotomies of flexors or extensors of the toes combined with capsulotomies of the underlying joints were needed before the deformities could be corrected. In all cases where there was no subluxation the result was sufficiently good to allow the patients to walk in shoes.

In 3 patients, partial resections of the basal phalanx (a modification of KELLER's operation) achieved their object. 5 toes had to be amputated (see p. 51).

9. Operations for flaccid limitation of extension at the hip

In 3 patients, neglect during earlier stages of treatment led to limitation of extension at the hip in cauda-equina lesions. All patients had been severely wounded and had been cachectic for years.

The sartorius and rectus femoris tendons formed sharp subcutaneous bands which often caused skin defects through friction by trousers.

Elongation was unnecessary where these muscles were completely paralysed. Tenotomy was done from a 4″ incision in a skin-crease well below the inguinal ligament. After division of the tendons, the legs were extended as far as possible. The anterior edge of fascia lata and adhesions between subcutaneous tissue and muscle were divided. No more drastic steps were needed.

Haemostasis has to be very accurate. In one patient, small haemotomata developed which had to be aspirated and cost the patient one additional week in bed. Correction of deformity left about 10 degrees of flexion in all patients. There was no further damage to the skin by friction.

10. Cases

Case I. Severe spastic flexion-contracture of the knee

In the majority of spastic contractures elimination of spasticity by the appropriate operation on muscle or tendon is sufficient to permit the gradual stretching of contracted ligaments and joint capsules by continuous maintenance of the corrected position and passive stretching by the physiotherapist.

Cases in which radical operations on capsule and ligaments become necessary, are rare. In such cases it is difficult to maintain post-operatively full correction of the deformity without causing ischaemic skin defects which may spoil the success of the operation.

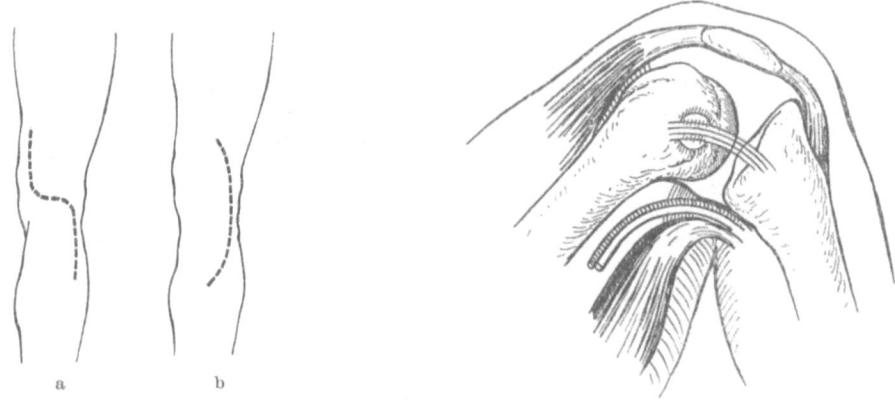

Fig. 12   Fig. 13

Fig. 12a u. b. a) Severe spastic flexion contracture of knee 1. Bajonett Incision. b) Flaccid flexion contracture of knee. Crescent incision

Fig. 13. Severe spastic flexion contracture of knee 2. Extent of adhesions and contractures (see text)

In a 34-year-old very muscular man with an incomplete, extremely spastic lesion below T. 11, we found an acute-angle flexion contracture of the knee. I planned to divide all limiting structures and exposed the lower third of the back of the thigh, the back of the knee and the upper third of the leg by a bayonet incision, the transverse part of which ran in the flexor crease.

The following pathology was found:

1. The skin had lost all elasticity and was firmly bound to the subcutaneous tissue.

2. The subcutaneous tissue had been converted into a hard fibrous mass, adherent both to skin and to the superficial fascia. These adhesions extended about 6″ proximally and distally from the flexor crease.

3. The superficial fascia was adherent to the muscles, the superficial flexors.

4. The tibial and peroneal nerves had to be shelled out of mantles of hard fibrous fat.

5. The popliteal vessels were so fixed by a similar fibrous block, the indurated gliding pad of fat, that they had to be carefully dissected out before they would slide again with movement of the joint.

6. The origins of the gastrocnemius showed extreme thickening of the fascia propria and were split transversely. The posterior capsule showed obliteration of its transverse folds and the posterior pouch by adhesions. After the capsule was transversely divided, the joint could be extended to 150 degrees, but it was clear that a further double-lock now prevented further extension.

7. Both collateral ligaments, which normally slide over their bursae behind the epicondyles of the femur, had been fixed in this position by adhesions around and within the bursae and had to be freed by blunt dissection. Only now did another 20 degrees of extension become possible.

After the most careful haemostasis, the skin, which had been widely mobilised, could just be made to meet with the knee in optimal extension. It was sutured with wire (gauge 36) and a thickly padded extension plaster-splint was applied over the *extensor* surface of the knee.

As expected, the skin-sutures cut out, the skin edges parted for nearly 2″ and healing by granulation, without signs of infection, took seven weeks. The patient could now stand and walk. Three years later, the result had been maintained.

The extent and multiplicity of the adhesions and shrinkage in this extreme case show us where we have to look for the causes of unsatisfactory results in less severe contractures, and how at times our "routine operations" barely touch the fringe of the problem.

Case II. Severe flaccid flexion-contracture of both knee joints

A further case of severe flexion-contracture, bilateral this time, occurred in the flaccid paralysis of a patient who had had a severe poliomyelitis. Treatment was further complicated by the fact that this was a young giant, 6' 7" tall, who fitted into no bed and had to flex his hips and knees in order to be at all comfortable He arrived five years after the start of his illness, asking to be enabled to stand. In order to try whether I could avoid delay in healing of the skin, I used on one side a 15" crescent-incision (see Fig. 12b).

Adhesions, though severe, were much less extensive than in Case I. and did not fix vessels and nerves. The skin healed by first intention.

The result was not perfect, since about 10 degrees of fixed flexion remained and passive extension exercises were too painful. The patient himself was very satisfied and stood with plaster-shells.

In this case, I made the serious mistake of operating without starting transfusion with the anaesthetic. His haemoglobin level had been 92% and only moderate bleeding occurred during operation. Suddenly he collapsed. An immediate saline-drip followed by emergency blood-transfusion had to be given before he recovered.

Case III. Severe flaccid extension contracture of the knee joints

A different mistake, this time in assessing the state of circulation in the skin, spoiled the result in another patient with poliomyelitis in whom we found severe extension contracture of both knees. Curiously enough, this was the result of deliberate planning by an earlier surgeon who hoped that it would enable the patient to walk without calipers. The surgeon's error consisted in not anticipating that a paralysed patient with extension contractures of the knees finds them a grave disadvantage for life in a wheelchair. (See next chapter.)

This patient asked for an improvement in flexion of his knees, so that he would be able to sit comfortably in his wheelchair and to turn it in a narrow space.

X-ray films showed the bony elements of the joint to be normal. The joint was opened from a long anterior incision and very massive adhesions in the joint-space and superior pouch were removed. After excision of the patella a long Z-elongation of the quadriceps tendon was carried out, permitting right-angle flexion of the knee.

Postoperatively, the thickly-bandaged leg was positioned in 60 degrees of flexion at the knee. Within a few days the skin over the patellar bed became ischaemic and sloughed in a circle of about 3" diameter. Even after the knee was extended, healing took several months and the extension-contracture recurred.

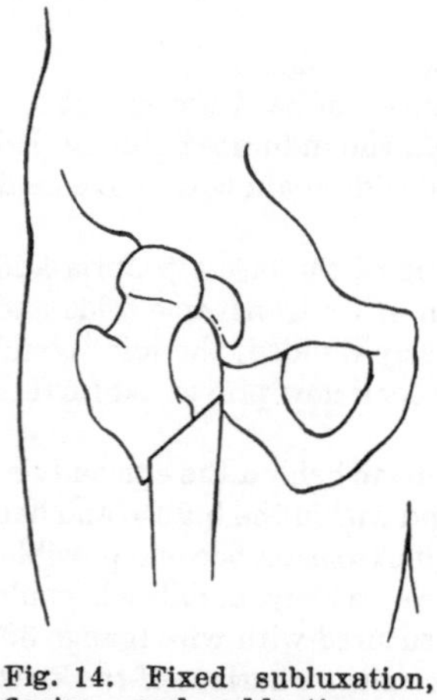

Fig. 14. Fixed subluxation, flexion- and adduction-contracture of hip. Deformity corrected by pertrochanteric osteotomy

Case IV. Severe adduction and flexion contracture of the hip with fixed subluxation

In a man aged 35, who was admitted two years after transverse myelitis in a state of extreme neglect and whose paralysis had largely recovered, an intertrochanteric osteotomy was needed to correct the position of the limb. This operation was only one incident in a four-year treatment of most extensive pressure sores and other contractures.

For the last six years, he has been walking with elbow-crutches and doing a full day's work.

B. Arthroplasty for extension-ankylosis of the knee-joint

(author's modification of the arthroplasty of Hass)

Occasionally we see patients who, owing to serious mismanagement, have contracted unilateral or bilateral ankylosis of the knee in extension.

a) Indication

In the patient without paralysis, we might prefer a painless, stable, stiff joint to a painful, unstable, mobile one, but to the paraplegic this ankylosis means a serious hindrance in his active life. He cannot turn his wheelchair in a narrow space; he cannot open doors or sit close to a desk or bench, and he cannot drive his car without expensive adjustments.

The patients themselves urged us to try to restore their knee-joints so that they could put their feet on the foot-rests of their chairs.

In no case was it easy to decide whether one should do what they wanted. Nothing was then known about the chances of arthroplasties in paralysed limbs. And while pain or flailness were not likely to endanger the result, the dangers of haemorrhage from large new bone-surfaces created without tourniquet in paralysed limbs, was something one could not ignore. The possibility of a re-ankylosis had also to be seriously considered.

b) Technique of the operation

The writer has experience of seven arthroplasties in five paraplegic patients. I used the technique described first by Hass (1925, 1930, 1944), because it is physiologically and mechanically sound. In one important detail I differed from his technique. Hass used interposition of fat — or fascia — sheets which, during his earlier work, was still considered essential. I knew that any foreign material, be it fat, fascia, metal or plastic, would endanger success and be eliminated. But I also felt that a more reliable result might be achieved with the help of an attractive idea of Stamm's. Stamm (1942) suggested that the post-operative haematoma within the new joint should be divided into two separate layers of fibrin to cover the new surfaces, by putting light traction on the leg a few days after the operation. In my material, this suggestion has produced satisfactory results. A new problem, specific to paraplegics, demanded a new solution. Three of our patients had, in addition to the ankylosis of the knee itself, a separate ankylosis of the patella on a stalk growing from the femoral surface. The skin over this fixed patella consisted of a tissue paper scar following earlier pressure sores. This meant that if one excised the patella, one would be left with a large skin-defect, which promised to become quite a problem. A solution was found in preserving a thin slice of patella attached to the skin and resecting the other 4/5 ths underneath it. However, two newly shaped bony surfaces were now facing each other and synostosis was likely to occur between them. I decided to detach the quadriceps tendon at the tibial tuberosity, to reverse it upwards, between the bone-surfaces, and to fix it with a few wire sutures near the upper pole of the patella.

In our first case, where apart from the ankylosis, there were periarticular ossifications, a synostosis recurred at the lateral edge of the patellar slice. In the two other joints the method worked well.

All patients in whom an arthroplasty had to be considered owed their ankylosis either to treatment in a plaster-bed with complete lack of passive movements, or to septic arthritis under pressure sores.

The first patient had spent four years and three months in a plaster-bed extending from his shoulders to his toes. Another patient with incomplete quadriplegia after subarachnoid haemorrhage and operation for an aneurysm of a cerebral artery had had no physiotherapy.

The other three patients had up to thirteen pressure sores each, of which some had entered their knee-joints and led to ankylosis. That the urinary tract of these patients was severely infected is understood. The second patient, on whom I operated ten years ago, died four years later of uraemia. The first and last patients needed bilateral arthroplasty. The ankylosis was fibrous in the second patient but bony in all others.

In the first and fourth case, periarticular ossification complicated the operation, in the first, third and fifth the stalk-ankylosis of the patella.

In the third patient, my modified operation was the third attempt at arthroplasty. Another surgeon had twice tried excision of the joint which did not achieve its object and left a massive calcified haematoma around the popliteal vessels. In the fourth patient, the other knee and both hips were also ankylosed (see next chapter).

In the fifth patient, both legs were also rotated inward owing to ectopic ossification at the hips. This was corrected by outward rotation at the knee obtained by cutting the new joint-surfaces obliquely. The feet, which before were severely inward rotated, were now standing parallel on the footrest. Instability due to stretching of the collateral ligaments was surprisingly small.

In all operations, a mobile joint was produced. Its range was unsatisfactory in the first case after three years, and in the fourth case after four months. The remaining five joints regained the desired flexion range.

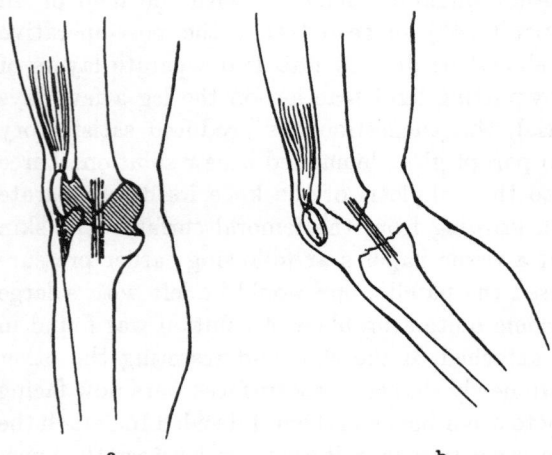

a   b

Fig. 15 a u. b. a) Ankylosis in extension of knee with stalk-ankylosis of patella. Shaping of new joint surfaces and extent of excision of bone. Note: subtotal excision of patella. b) Ankylosis in extension of the knee 2. New joint-surfaces (after HASS). The patellar ligament is slung up between patellar slice and new surface of femur

In no case was a tourniquet used. The first patient needed no anaesthetic.

The joint was opened from a long anterolateral or anteromedial incision taking care not to incise through scars.

The new joint-surfaces were shaped and the sub-total excision of the patella was carried out as shown in the drawings.

Haemostasis with diathermy was satisfactory, in spite of the production of large coagulated surfaces. The incision was closed with two layers of accurate interrupted wire sutures (gauges 40 and 36) and, after the dressing, a woolmantle was applied with an elastic bandage. The knee was positioned in slight flexion and passive movement started by the surgeon on the second day.

c) Postoperative Treatment

On the third day, skin-traction over a woolmantle was applied with a weight of 4 lbs.

Effusion occurred during the first weeks and in all cases increased during the third and fourth week, without any local or general signs of infection. A sterile secretion of blood-stained synovia developed which persisted for about two to three weeks, by which time the opening had healed under simple sterile dressings.

Passive movements were restricted during this period but continued every day. On average, the patients were able to sit in the chair, with their feet on the footrest, within two months. Only in one knee of the last patient did a synovial fistula recur after eight months; once more, this healed spontaneously within three weeks.

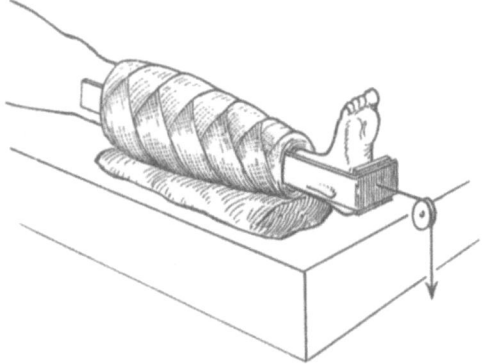

Fig. 16. Skin-Traction. Note: traction-plaster applied over thick woolmantle, fixed to skin only over tibial condyles. Leg on pillow, heel free from pressure

The following table contains details and results:

Table 21. *Arthroplasty of the knee-joint. Results*

No.	Neurological Symptomatology	No. of Operations	Length of follow-up	Range of movement
1	T. 12, complete, flaccid.	2	4 years	175/125 degrees 175/130 degrees
2	L. 1, incomplete, flaccid.	1	2½ years	175/105 degrees
3	T. 5, complete spastic.	1	9 years	180/100 degrees
4	Cerebral Aneurysm normal	1	4 months	175/130 degrees
5	T. 6, complete, flaccid.	2	1 year	180/90 degrees 180/90 degrees

Summary

In cases of ankylosis of the knee in extension, the restoration of a flexion range is important for the rehabilitation of the paraplegic. His return to work may depend on the success of the arthroplasty. The final result depends largely on the correct timing and degree of passive movements after the operation. The surgeon himself should carry out this treatment during the first few weeks.

C. Operations for para-articular ectopic ossification

Table 22. *Statistics*

Number of patients:	8
Number of operations:	11
(at the hip joint:	9
at the elbow joint:	2)

Neurological symptomatology		Complete	Incomplete
	Cervical	—	3
	T. 1—5	2	—
	T. 6—10	1	—
	T. 11 and below	1	—
	Cerebral		1
		4	4
		8	

Para-articular ossification is not uncommon in the paraplegic. Neurogenic ectopic bone formation has been described by RIEDEL (1883), EICHHORST (1895), KOENIG (1906), POETZL (1908) KUETTNER (1908) and others.

The first detailed descriptions we owe to Prof. and Mme. DÉJÉRINE and to CEILLIER (1918, 1919 and 1920).

More recently, ABRAMSON (1948), ABRAMSON and KAMBERG (1949), NISSEN-LIE (1953), BORS (1955), BERNSON (1956), EBEL (1956), FINKELMAN (1956), FINKLE (1956), ARMSTRONG-RESSY (1957), LODGE (1957), BÉNASSY (1957, 1960, 1961, 1963), COMARR (1958), STREET (1958), STEHMANN (1959), BURKE (1960), STEPANEK and STEPANEK (1960), DAMANSKI (1961), FREEHAFER, LOWRIE and LINKE (1961), MACEWEN (1962) and HARDY and DICKSON (1963) have published clinical, radiological and pathological observations. (For further sources, see STEHMANN, and HARDY and DICKSON.)

Pathology

The contributions of BÉNASSY and his collaborators contain biochemical data which point to a severe disturbance of the Co_2 exchange in the blood of paralysed limbs with ectopic ossification and represent a new approach to the elucidation of the pathogenesis. The former hypotheses, assuming as causes repeated trauma leading to multiple haematomata in muscle, and abnormalities in the histochemistry of bone, have not found acceptance.

The two forms of ectopic ossification, which must clinically be kept apart, have not been sufficiently distinguished in some of the literature. Ectopic ossification around osteomyelitic or septic arthritic foci underlying pressure-sores forms one group. The other represents ossification in the soft parts in the absence of infection.

Here we shall deal, with one exception, only with operations for the removal of ankylosing ossifications of the second group. One of the cases shown by NISSEN-LIE (1953) and the case shown by HARDY and DICKSON (1963), who report satisfactory operative results in seven further cases without giving details, belong with certainty to the "aseptic" group.

Methods of operation

1. Para-articular Pseudarthrosis

a) Technique of the operation

(patients 2, 3, 4. Table 23)

A segment, 1 to 3″ long, of the shaft of the femur below the minor trochanter was excised. The proximal end of the distal fragment was so shaped that only an edge of bone opposed the distal end of the proximal shaft. On both sides I sealed the bone-ends with layers of periosteum stripped off the excised fragment.

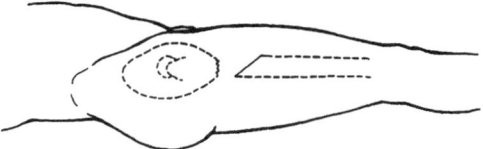

Fig. 17. Para-articular ossification at hip 1. Para-articular pseudarthrosis. Shaping the distal shaft of femur

Following this operation flexion to 90 degrees in the new joint was possible and remained satisfactory for a few weeks. After two months, however, extensive new ossification occurred which, in one of the three patients, permitted flexion to only 50 degrees three years later.

In the other two patients, complete ankylosis recurred. The bilateral operation on a patient with ankylosis of both hips and both knees which followed an operation for aneurysm of a cerebral artery and incomplete quadriparesis was a complete failure. An unusual finding in this case was a rise of the serum alkaline phosphatase to 60 King-Armstrong units 100/ml.

The last patient had an ankylosis of the hip following septic arthritis. Although the joint was not opened, a sinus formed after the operation and had not closed two years later. When seen a few months ago, the sinus had healed. There had been a fracture through the reossified zone and a 90° flexion-range resulted.

2. Excision of the ectopic bone

a) Technique of the operation

(patients 1, 5, 6, 7, 8. Table 23)

Five operations at the hip and two at the elbow consisted of the excision of all, or most, of the ectopic bone in those cases where a short distal segment had to be left in situ, in order to avoid damaging the femoral vessels. In two patients

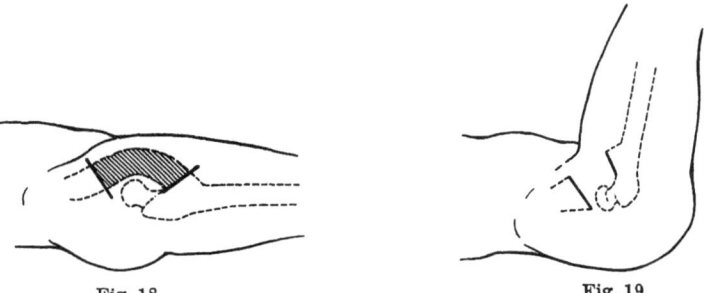

Fig. 18   Fig. 19

Fig. 18. Para-articular ossification at hip 2. Excision of ossified Iliopsoas

Fig. 19. Flexion-range after excision

(Table 23, No. 1 and 7), bilaterally in one case, blocks of bone measuring 8″ in length and up to 3″ in depth and width, had to be removed from the front of the hips. Haemostasis was as thorough as possible and a drain was left in situ for three days. All incisions healed promptly, but in the first patient late infection of the second hip developed. Both joints re-ankylosed. No sinus formed and the patient has worked at home for the last six years. The other patient, who had a massive ossification of the iliopsoas on one side is, as far as I know, the only instance in which a single severe local trauma produced a large haematoma in front of the hip and damaged the hip-joint itself. She had been a paraplegic for ten years (complete flaccid lesion below T. 3) when her foot was caught in the carpet of her car while she was trying to turn herself into the seat of her wheelchair. A large swelling in front of the hip led to complete ankylosis within six months. Nine years later, I operated and removed very nearly the whole of the ossified mass. There was a bony bridge between the mass and the neck of femur which rendered opening of the joint necessary.

One year later, the radiograph showed several calcified shadows in the neighbourhood of the joint, but a free flexion movement to 90 degrees has been maintained.

Two further patients (Table 23, No. 5 and 6) had ossifications of the anterolateral muscles of the hip without involvement of the iliopsoas. Ankylosis was complete. In both cases, excision led to a freely mobile joint. Two and three years after the operation, the flexion-angle was 80⁰ and 90⁰ respectively. Success in these last three operations may be due to the application of a new idea of Dr. GUTTMANN. He suggested that, after complete haemostasis, the cut bone-surfaces and surrounding soft parts should be dabbed and injected with a sterile solution of 10% Formalin. This corresponded to the well known method used for the prevention of the development or recurrence of neuromata after peripheral nerve-injuries or amputations (GUTTMANN and MEDAWAR 1942).

Dr. GUTTMANN took part in two operations and carried this treatment out himself.

This small number of patients does not, of course, permit an assessment of the value of this method. Further experience will show in which cases we can count on success.

The patient (Table 23, No. 8) with bilateral ossification in the distal triceps brachii had an incomplete lesion below C 3—4 due to trauma. He had also suffered for 30 years from extensive psoriasis. The ankylosis were complete, but radiologically the joints were not involved. At operation, it was impossible to find a dividing line between humerus and ectopic bone and the joints had to be opened. Formalin was used in one operation. In both joints ankylosis recurred.

b) Postoperative treatment

In cases such as these, postoperative control of blood-pressure and haemoglobin-level is particularly important. The leg should be positioned in about 40⁰ flexion. All passive movement should be carried out by the surgeon himself for the first few weeks.

The critical period is the first two months. Clinical findings and radiographs do not always tally. The range of movement may be much better than shadows in the film would suggest. If the surgeon acquires the 'feel' of the movement of the joint, he will know long before the next radiograph what he can expect.

Table 23. *Operations for para-articular ectopic ossification. Results*

No.	Cause of paraplegia	Site of ankylosis	Method of operation	Result	Follow up
1.	Myelitis, C 6, incomplete	Both hips	Excision	Failure, infection	8 years
2.	Vascular cause, C 7, complete	One hip	Pseudarthrosis	50° flexion	3 years
3.	Cerebral, incomplete	Both hips	Pseudarthrosis	Failure after 4 months	
4.	Epidural abscess, C 6, incomplete	One hip (old sepsis)	Pseudarthrosis	Flare-up of infection	2 years
5.	Fracture T 6 vertebra T 6, complete	One hip	Excision and formalin	80° free flexion	2 years
6.	Fracture T 12 vertebra L 1, complete	One hip	Excision and formalin	90° free flexion	3 years
7.	Myelitis, T 3, complete	One hip (local trauma)	Excision and formalin	90° free flexion	1 year
8.	Fracture C 3/4 vertebra C 4, incomplete	Both elbows	Excision; formalin on one side	Failure	6 months

Summary

"Neurogenic" ectopic ossification may demand operative treatment, but only if it has led to complete or almost complete ankylosis at the hip- or elbow-joints, when it seriously impairs the independence of the patient.

Excision of the greater part of the ossified mass is the method of choice, recurrence and infection are the main risks. GUTTMANN's formalin method may be helpful in the prevention of recurrence.[1]

D. Operation for septic arthritis of the hip-joint

Table 24. *Neurological symptomatology*

Level	Complete	Incomplete
Cervical	1	1
T. 1—5	3	1
T. 6—10	2	—
T. 11 and below	—	1
	6	3

9 patients

[1] In future reports it would seem desirable that cases are separated into those where calcification occurred with or without infection of the underlying joint from pressure sores. Accurate measurement of the pre- and postoperative range of movement and assessment of results not before the end of the first year after the operation would help in developing the most reliable technique.

Table 25. *Time-gap between start of paraplegia and operation for septic arthritis of the hip*

Years	Patients
3	1
6	2
9	1
10	1
11	2
14	1
17	1
	9

Many patients arrived at the Centre many years after the start of their paraplegia.

They were in a dreadful state; cachectic, anaemic and toxic, with eight, ten or twelve pressure sores, severe infection of the urinary tract and the typical contractures of early mismanagement. Often they were still young and intelligent, with full insight into their situation.

After blood-transfusions, turning, antibiotics and active retraining had transformed them from hopeless into hopeful people, there remained, with some of them, a difficult problem. Years of osteomyelitis beneath the sores over ischium or trochanter had produced septic invasion of the hip-joint. Both the head and neck of femur and the acetabulum were partially destroyed.

Pathology: In the paraplegie this creeping infection is easily overlooked. There is no pain. The raised temperature is attributed to the simultaneous infection of the urinary tract. We have had patients in whom the destruction of the joint was far advanced yet who, before arrival, had never had a radiograph taken of this region.

This most severe bone — and joint — infection may even die out by itself and heal, after destruction of the acetabulum and upper end of femur, leading to a pathological dislocation. In other patients, infection threatens life, if not immediately then over the years. Amyloid degeneration of kidneys and other organs has to be expected.

We have seen a number of cases in which an attempt was made to remove the diseased bone via the pressure sore. In all of them this method led to relapse with a flare-up and further spread of the infection.

MILLER (1956), STREET (1958), STEPANEK and STEPANEK (1960), SCHNEIDER and KRUG (1960) and FREEHAFER, LOWRY and LINKE (1961) have reported on cases and operations. Their results are not convincing.

a) Technique of the operation

I decided to approach the joint via healthy tissue, to remove diseased bone as radically as possible and to use the pressure-sore as a channel for drainage only. In nine patients with operations on twelve hips, this method has proved effective.

If one excises the proximal end of the femur as far down as 2″ below the minor trochanter, a new problem arises. The femur, and with it the whole limb, has now lost all control of rotation. The leg may roll 90⁰ or more inwards or outwards and exerts a diagonal screw-effect on the femoral vessels which seriously interferes with circulation.

Attempts to prevent this rolling with a slipper splint were successful, but tended to produce pressure-sores on the dorsum pedis and heel which, in spite of daily inspection, could not always be prevented and took months to heal.

In my last two patients, I have used the un-operated leg as a splint for the operated one. The "swaddle splint" has worked well.

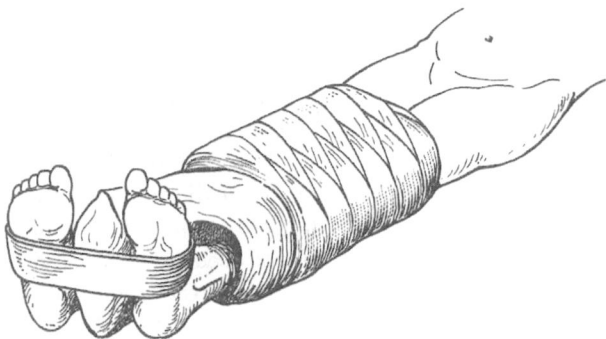

Fig. 20. Operation for septic arthritis of the hip-joint 1. The swaddle-splint. Pillows between and around both legs, held with elastic bandages. Feet secured by thickly padded elastic bandage

The patient's general state must be as good as possible, with a haemoglobin level of 100% and blood-urea near the normal. He is positioned on his back. Femur and hip-joint are approached from the front. The long SMITH-PETERSEN approach is very suitable.

The shaft of the femur is exposed at the level of the trochanter minor. The extensive mass of fibrosed and calcified soft parts is dissected and split centripetally.

The circumflex vessels are, where possible, dissected and tied before division. The femoral vessels are protected and retracted by two ringhandle-spikes introduced between them and the medial surface of the femur.

Blunt, patient dissection, with the occasional aid of the osteotome, frees the mutilated, often crumbling, proximal end of the femur up to the joint-capsule. This is opened with a long incision, so that the destroyed acetabulum can be well displayed. At the distal end of the skin incision the shaft of femur is now transversely divided with saw and osteotome.

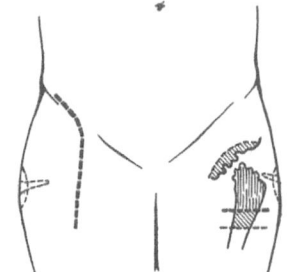

Fig. 21. On right: Smith-Petersens' anterior approach. Note: posterolateral sore and sinus. On left: Extent of resection of femur and acetabulum

The cut surfaces are examined. The marrow-cavity may be closed and eburnised indicating that here osteomyelitis has died out and sealed off. The bone may, however, crumble, and the marrow-cavity may contain a mixture of degenerated marrow and pus. In this case, the marrow-cavity has to be cleared with a sharp spoon and the proximal end of the distal shaft of the femur resected further, until healthy-looking bone is encountered.

Appearances on radiographs are unreliable guides.

The distal end of the proximal femur-segment is now gripped with strong bone-forceps and, proceeding proximally, is shelled out until it can be removed in one piece. Haemostasis follows every step. The wide-open, and now almost empty, cavity shows laterally the inner entrance into the sinus of the pressure-sore and medially the remnants of the acetabulum, often masked by osteophytes. All diseased tissue is removed from here without accidentally entering the true pelvis.

Necrotic synovialis and the walls of abscess-cavities are excised, together with calcified parts of fibrotic muscle, ligaments and joint-capsule. Some fibrotic coat is left in situ to serve as an internal splint.

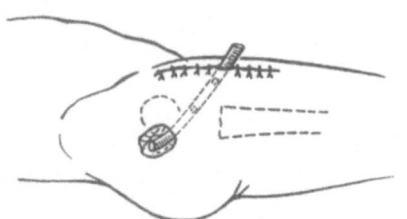

Fig. 22. Lateral view at end of operation. Note: bone-gap. Drainage-tube from anterior incision through joint- space to sinus

The large cavity is washed out thoroughly with warm saline to remove all detritus.

A drainage tube, about 12" long, with an inner diameter of 1 cm. and with side-holes distributed over its middle third, is introduced into the cavity in such a way that its anterior end will be led out through the skin-incision. The posterior end is led out, from inside outward, through the pressure-sore sinus.

After once more making sure of good haemostasis, the capsule, fascia and skin are closed with interrupted wire sutures (gauge 36) in two layers. The drain protrudes between two skin-sutures. Skin-adaptation has to be very accurate.

Two separate dressings of thick gauze under elastoplast cover the operation-wound and pressure-sore.

During the operation, which lasts 1½ to 2 hours, two to three pints of blood are transfused. The wide opening of the joint will produce collapse, unless the anaesthetist has speeded up the transfusion in good time. Transfusion, followed if necessary by saline and glucose drips, continues during the operation day and the following night, if the patient is still unable to drink. Further blood-transfusions may be needed within the next two or three days.

b) Postoperative treatment

Control of pulse and blood-pressure has to be very thorough for the first few days. Dressings are changed daily. For three days, the drain is washed through from the front with warm saline, followed by instillation of a solution of 5% Penicillin or Chloromycetin. On the fourth day, the posterior end od the drain is pulled down until the anterior end disappears under the suture line. One or two secondary skin-sutures complete the closure of the incision.

During the following days, the drain is washed out from below and every other day it is shortened by about one inch. The choice of rinsing-solution is determined by bacteriological and sensitivity tests.

The skin incision will be healed by the twelfth day and the sutures are removed. The sinus is kept open, but the original drain is gradually replaced by thinner tubes introduced for shorter distances.

Within a few days of the operation, the surgeon flexes the limb once or twice daily to 90 degrees without permitting undue rotation. This fulfils two important purposes:

1. It acts as a pump, helping to remove fluid and detritus from the cavity.

2. It helps to shape the fibrinous cover over the cut bone. This soft network will later calcify and form new bone as a scar which, as we have seen, may even copy the shape of a femoral neck.

In all my cases, the sores were healed within three to eight weeks after the operation.

c) Complications and failures

In my second case, infection extended so far distally into the shaft of femur that I did not dare to resect it all. On this side soft-part abscesses recurred twice during the first two years, leading to re-admission, local conservative treatment and blood-transfusions. The operation was done five years ago and the last abscess formed three years ago. When seen a few months ago, there was no sign of a recurrence and the patient was in excellent general health. In my last case, mine was a second operation, after an unsuccessful attempt elsewhere. After one year, there has been a return of a narrow fistula[1]. I may not have excised enough of the very widely infected soft tissue. All the other patients are in good general health and have shown no signs of recurrence (see following table).

Table 26. *Operation for septic arthritis of the hip-joint. Results*

No.	Cause of paraplegia	Age	Result	Period of follow-up
1.	Tumor, T 6 complete	21	Bilateral, healed, works full-time	5½ years
2.	Fracture T 3/4, T 4 complete	32	Bilateral, healed, unilateral abscess 3 years ago. Housewife	4½ years
3.	Tumor, T 3/4 complete	41	Unilateral, healed	4 years
4.	Fracture C 3/4, C 5 complete	21	Unilateral, healed	3 years
5.	D. S., C 5 complete	31	Bilateral, healed	2 years
6.	Fracture T 9/10, T 10 complete	43	Unilateral, healed, at work	2 years
7.	Epidural abscess T 5 complete	22	Unilateral, healed, at work	1 year
8.	Tumour T 5 complete	21	Unilateral, healed, works full-time	1 year
9.	Myelitis T 12 incomplete	23	Unilateral, sinus.	1 year

Summary

An operative and post-operative method of treatment for advanced septic arthritis of the hip-joint of paraplegics is described which has proved satisfactory on 12 occasions. Long term results show that a condition which endangers life can be eliminated, and that the majority of patients were able to return to work.

---

[1] This sinus closed spoutaneously since and has not reopened for one year.

E. Fractures of the long bones

We have by now sufficient experience in the indications and treatment of fractures of the long bones in the paraplegic to allow us to define the differences, in principle, compared with those of the "normal".

Healing of fractures in the paraplegic presents no problem. They unite well and rapidly (HALL et. al. 1953, GUTTMANN 1954 and BORS 1955). However, the technique of conservative treatment is governed by the need to prevent pressure-sores, and operation is permissible only where, as far as is humanly possible, we can guarantee prevention of infection.

All operations for fractures on long bones are done under general anaesthesia and without a tourniquet.

There are two main groups of fractures, the associated fractures and the late fractures in old paraplegics. Each group raises its own problems.

It also makes a difference whether the fracture occurs in a paralysed or a non-paralysed limb.

We have seen 74 patients with 82 fractures of the first group, more than 100 patients belonging to the second group, and other patients showing the results of treatment elsewhere.

COMARR, HUTCHINSON and Bors (1959, 1962) have published large statistics which include not only fractures of the long bones but also other fractures. Fractures associated with the spinal injury were treated in the hospitals to which their patients were first admitted, and, in these cases, the authors had to rely on records. In their treatment of secondary fractures, they emphasize the need for the prevention of pressure-sores and accept, if need be, some malalignment. EICHENHOLTZ (1963) comes to the same conclusion in his report of 32 fractures. The results, which he describes, of treating fractures of the limbs of paraplegics with the conservative and operative methods used for non-paralysed patients, tell a grim story.

1. Associated fractures of the long bones

Table 27. *Statistics*

	Upper Limb. bilateral compound				Lower Limb. bilateral compound		
Humerus	12	—	2	Femur	13	1	5
Forearm	15	1	5	Tibia-Fibula	15	—	6
Wrist	14	3	—	Ankle	13	3	3
Fractures	41	4	7	*Fractures*	41	4	14
Patients	*37*			*Patients*	*37*		

The majority of the patients were admitted to us only shortly after primary treatment of the fractures. The numbers for upper and lower limbs are identical. Only one patient had a fracture of the radius combined with a fracture of the femur. Fractures were more often compound in the lower limb.

Of other fractures, those of the ribs and the skull were most common. Pelvis, scapula, jaw and nose were more often involved than the clavicle; fractures of the tarsal bones and toes were more common than fractures of carpal bones and fingers. Fractures of the sternum were found only in four cases of fracture-dislocations of T. 3/4, T. 4/5 and T. 5/6. With this exception, there were no standard combinations, neither according to the type of accident, nor in relation to the level of the spinal injury.

There were two cases of traumatic dislocation of the hip. Lesions of peripheral nerves were seen only in the upper limb (plexus paralysis 4, radial paralysis 3).

Associated fractures are fairly common but in Britain particularly as a result of motor-cycle accidents. Compared with the spinal injury and other severe injuries, they often constitute a minor evil, the treatment of which may have to wait. The question of priorities has to be clearly answered.

Priorities. The patient may not only be in severe surgical and spinal shock, he may also often have concussion with or without fracture of the skull, injuries to nose or jaw, fractures of ribs, clavicle, scapula and sternum, with or without pneumo- and haemothorax, tears of the mediastinum or diaphragm, or ruptures of abdominal organs or kidneys.

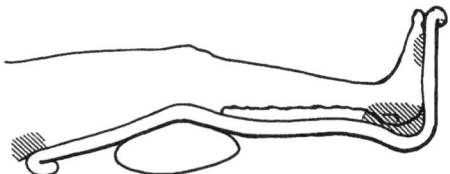

Fig. 23. Kramer leg-splint. Note: thick padding, overhanging edges, double padding under calf, Heel free. main danger areas for pressure-sores: ▪

On admission, he may be unconscious. Consequently, the spinal injury may often be overlooked; this may be difficult to avoid and paraplegia may not be suspected even after he recovers. The most urgent surgical measures, after treatment for shock and massive blood-transfusions, will be devoted to haemostasis in skull, chest and abdomen.

If, under such circumstances, paralysis is discovered early and turning is instituted, pressure-sores can be prevented. Catheterisation, under strict surgical asepsis, can often be postponed for 24 hours. Aspirations of a tension-pneumothorax or haemothorax are compatible with turning. Where mechanical ventilation of the lungs is needed, the patient can, at least, be lifted two-hourly, the sheets can be adjusted and his back and heels inspected and protected by suitably arranged sponge-rubber cushions.

While general shock is being treated and haemostasis achieved, limb-fractures have to be immobilised on Kramer splints, thickly padded.

Displacement at the fracture-site may have to wait for reduction until the acute danger to the patient's life has passed.

In such cases, it may take a week before one can plan the treatment of these fractures having proper regard for all complicating factors.

Conservative treatment. In contrast to the upper limb, fractures of the femur and leg can, in most cases, be treated conservatively, on thickly-padded Kramer or plaster splints, with inspection for the prevention of pressure-sores daily at first and later on alternate days. Traction (see Fig. 16, p. 29) may also be needed. On turning, the leg has to be moved in complete alignment with the body. Even compound fractures heal well and in good position with this method. Neurological examination will tell, within a few weeks, whether recovery from paralysis is likely. In any case, fractures have to be treated in such a way that the patient will be able to stand and walk as normally as possible.

Healing time is normal or, with the help from the large fracture-haematoma, may even be shorter than normal. A period of three to four months in bed is needed; this is not much longer than is required for consolidation of the spinal injury.

Fracture-healing and spasticity. The fear that spasms might interfere seriously with fracture healing is hardly ever justified. After the first three weeks, when in most transverse cord lesions spasticity begins, fibrous pre-callus is generally strong enough to prevent displacement by spasms.

Nailing of the femur can be defended, when the general condition of the patient permits. Splints which immobilise the proximal end of the femur, or a hip spica, cannot be used because they produce sores over the tuber ischii or trochanter. One must realise, however, that the main effect of nailing is some easing of nursing the patient; it is not required to ensure healing of the fracture. And even a nail may fail.

Case V. Conservative treatment of threatened non-union of nailed femur

A man aged 20 had a severe motor-cycle accident, resulting in a fracture-dislocation of L. 1 vertebra with complete paraplegia below L. 1 and fractures of the mid-shafts of both femora, simple on the right, compound on the left side. In his first hospital he was treated for shock and with Küntscher nails on both sides. On the right the nail fitted well. On the left the distal fragment partially slipped off.

Unfortunately, the paraplegia was entirely ignored. Two weeks later the patient was admitted to us with a sacral sore some 12" across and a haemoglobin-level of 50%.

Four weeks later his general condition was good, the pressure-sore was clean and granulating well and the wound over the left femur had healed. The distal fragment of the left femur, however, still moved freely and obliquely around the end of the nail. There was a gap between the fragments of more than 1", due to a loss of bone-substance at the time of the accident. Meanwhile we knew that paraplegia would remain complete and permanent.

The question was whether we should remove the nail because it did not fulfil its purpose and whether open reduction and fixation were indicated.

I made the attempt to push the distal fragment up the nail until the bone-ends were impacted, and maintained this position by a short anterior plaster splint wrapped on the thigh with elastic bandaging. In six weeks the fracture was firmly united. The one inch shortening was compensated for by a raised sole and heel.

Operative treatment. Associated fractures of the humerus and forearm pose a very different problem from fractures of the lower limb. In fractures of the humerus in the paraplegic, who has to remain in bed and be turned for three months, it is impossible to immobilise the fracture of the shaft of the humerus. An aeroplane splint would threaten the skin over the paralysed chest or abdomen.

Nevertheless, it is particularly important to have a perfect reduction of the humerus and to avoid all stiffness in shoulder, elbow or forearm. The arms will, after all, become weight-bearing limbs if paralysis of the legs does not recover.

a) Upper extremity: Early operations: Indications

Operative reduction and fixation of the humerus are indicated as soon as the general condition of the patient permits; usually at the end of the first or the beginning of the second week. I do not rely on nailing. In a patient lying in bed who has to be frequently turned, the danger of rotation of the distal fragment is too great to be prevented by a nail.

I prefer a four-hole vitallium plate which has done good service in two cases.

Case VI. Early open reduction and plating of the shaft of the humerus, in a case with radial palsy

In a patient aged 21 the fracture healed in near-perfect alignment in eight weeks. The radial palsy recovered completely. Paraplegia remained complete below L. 1.

This heavy young man has walked very well with calipers and elbow-crutches for the last five years. Range of movement of all joints remains normal.

Case VII. Early open reduction and plating of the comminuted shaft of the humerus, combined with plexus-paralysis

A man aged 28 with a complete cauda equina lesion below L. 1 after fracture-dislocation of L. 1 vertebra, a complete paralysis of the brachial plexus and a comminuted fracture of the shaft of the humerus on the same side, had a similar early operation in which, in addition, the third fragment was fixed with a separate screw.

Again the fracture healed within eight weeks, in perfect alignment. Unfortunately, there was no recovery of the plexus-paralysis or the cauda-equina lesion. Four and a half years later the patient is fit and can stand, but cannot use a crutch because of the plexus lesion.

What may happen, if early open fixation is not done, was demonstrated by a patient who was treated conservatively elsewhere. Pseudarthrosis resulted. After two bone grafting operations elsewhere, union occurred with severe deformity and an elbow which was so stiff that a crutch could not be used.

Even in cervical lesions, there may be a case for open fixation of a fractured humerus-shaft.

Fractures of the forearm: Indications. The reason for the best possible reduction and fixation are similarly strong in the forearm. The goal of treatment must be to maintain, not only full mobility of elbow and wrist, but also full pronation and supination.

Many fractures of either ulna or radius can be reduced and kept reduced by simple plaster-splints. In cervical lesions fractures of both bones of the forearm should also be treated conservatively. During the first three weeks some malalignment might temporarily be accepted. It may be corrected at that stage by gentle manipulation, if possible without anaesthetic, and will often lead to a good result.

The Monteggia fracture demands special measures. It should be treated by open reduction and plating or nailing. Two of our patients were operated on before admission. Reduction and result were disappointing. The stiff forearm was a serious drawback for the patients.

b) Upper extremity: Late operations: Indications

In rare instances one may have to accept severe displacement in the forearm for the time being, because the general condition of the patient does not permit anaesthesia.

Case VIII. Fracture of lower third of ulna combined with fracture-dislocation of T 8/9 vertebra, incomplete paraplegia and haemothorax, mediastinal tear and brain injury

This 29-year-old man was neither mentally nor physically fit enough for two months to permit removal of the distal fragment of the ulna which had healed in severe malalignment. After a further two months, the patient was able to walk well with elbow-crutches, without pain in his wrist.

Case IX. Fracture of both bones of the forearm on one side and of the ulna on the other side, combined with fracture-dislocation of C. 5/6, complete quadriplegia below C. 6 and haemothorax

A man aged 22 suffered in a motor-cycle accident a fracture-dislocation of C. 5/6 vertebrae with complete quadriplegia below C. 6.; he had a fracture of both bones of the forearm on one side, of the ulna alone on the other side, but a haemothorax and severe respiratory disturbance made any reduction impossible for the first two months.

Ten weeks after the accident, when he was fit, bone splinters were removed from the site of the double-fracture; removal of the malunited fragment was carried out on the other side. Both forearms now function well within the limits of the paralysis. The patient can support himself between parallel bars and can play table-tennis with the racket wrapped to his hand.

Two other young men had severe injuries at the wrist. Bilateral distal radial slipped epiphyses could only be reduced after many weeks because of a haemothorax. Reduction was incomplete but no growth-disturbance followed.

A comminuted fracture at the wrist produced a paresis of the median nerve. Removal of the compressing callus led to recovery which has been maintained for five years.

c) Lower extremity: Late operations: Indications

Occasionally it is necessary to postpone reduction and fixation of fractures in the lower limb, because of severe other complications.

Case X. Supracondylar fracture of femur. Limitation of knee-flexion

A man aged 58 sustained, in an accident at work, a fracture-dislocation of T. 8/9 vertebrae with complete and permanent paraplegia below T. 8. Paralysis remained flaccid.

A severe haemothorax and a flare-up of an old tuberculous infection rendered anaesthesia impossible. A supracondylar fracture reaching into the knee-joint healed in bad position so that flexion of the knee was reduced to 20 degrees. At operation four months after the accident, the callus was excised, the fracture reduced and the distal fragment fixed with a long screw.

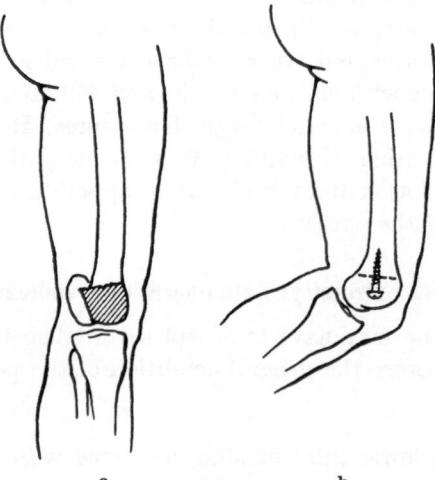

a   b

Fig. 24a u. b. Mal-union of supracondylar fracture of femur with limitation of knee-flexion. Late operation. Excision of callus, reduction and screw-fixation

Two months later the fracture had healed once more; extension of the knee was full, flexion was possible to 90 degrees and the foot could easily be put on the foot rest. The result has been maintained for two years.

Case XI. Comminuted fracture of tibial condyles. Limitation of knee-flexion

A man aged 31 with an incomplete cauda-equina lesion below L. 4 after fracture-dislocation of L. 1 vertebra suffered in addition a severe haemothorax and a comminuted fracture of the tibial condyles with much displacement. We had to wait for three months before we could reduce the fracture and fix it with screws. Again flexion to a right angle was restored; this patient walks with crutches. The result has been maintained for eighteen months.

In only two cases have we seen pseudarthrosis develop. The cause in the first case was overpulling of the fracture with 12 lbs. via a STEINMAN pin. In the second case a compound fracture was infected.

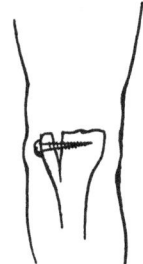

Fig. 25. Malunion of condylar fracture of tibia with limitation of knee-flexion. Late operation. Excision, partial reduction and screw-fixation

Case XII. Pseudarthrosis of femur. Plating and sliding graft

A man aged 45 with a broom stick spine after spondylosis suffered a motor-cycle accident. Permanent flaccid paraplegia below L. 1 followed a fracture-dislocation through the body of the 12th dorsal vertebra. There was also a transverse fracture of the midshaft of the femur.

He was admitted to us ten days after the accident when the fragments were shown to be distracted by 1½″ and the drillholes were infected. The pin was removed, traction reduced to four pounds and the leg treated on a Kramer-splint. Four months later some callus was visible, but there was also ample movement at the fracture-site. The marrow-cavity at both bone ends showed sealing off.

The findings at operation and the technique of fixation may be of interest.

Operation. The callus was exposed from a long antero-lateral incision. It consisted of a shell of calcified periosteum, some 8″ long, 3″ wide and more than 1″ deep, which contained a turbid, greyish-yellow fluid. This looked like pus but proved to be a sterile mixture of serum and bone marrow. Since the patient had always had a normal temperature, fixation of the fracture was undertaken.

The shaft of femur on both sides showed a raw irregular surface; the ends were in good alignment but were separated by an inch of fibrous scar tissue. On either side the marrow-cavity showed sealing off.

The technical problem was how to prevent refracture in a limb with a flaccid paralysis in which the distal extremity with its considerable weight had to be very firmly held. Some grafting too was required at this stage, if possible without taking bone from another incision.

The bone-ends were freshened and the marrow-cavities opened up. A long 8 hole Vitallium plate was placed laterally and fixed with three screws on each side of the fracture. The two holes nearest the fracture were not used.

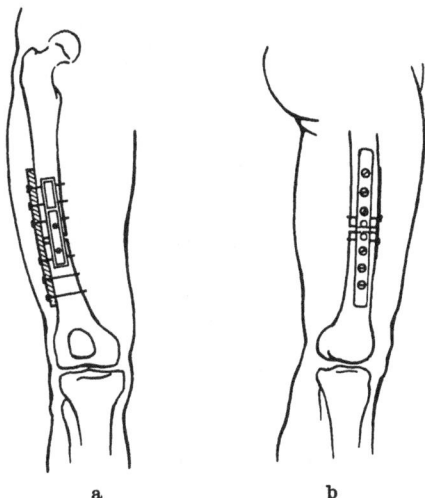

a   b

Fig. 26a u. b. Pseudarthrosis of femur. 1. Late operation. Excision of fibrous callus, opening-up of marrow cavities. Lateral 8 hole Vitallium plate. The 2 middle-holes are not used. 2. Anterior, strongly bevelled sliding-graft, fixed with 2 screws

A sliding-graft, with strongly-bevelled edges, was cut on the anterior surface and fixed across the fracture with two screws.

Healthy spongiosa from the marrow-cavities was packed around the fracture and the incision closed. Healing was undisturbed. Callus after four months was strong. Six months after the operation, the patient was able to stand. Again the result has proved satisfactory for eighteen months.

Case XIII. Pseudarthrosis of the tibia. Sliding graft

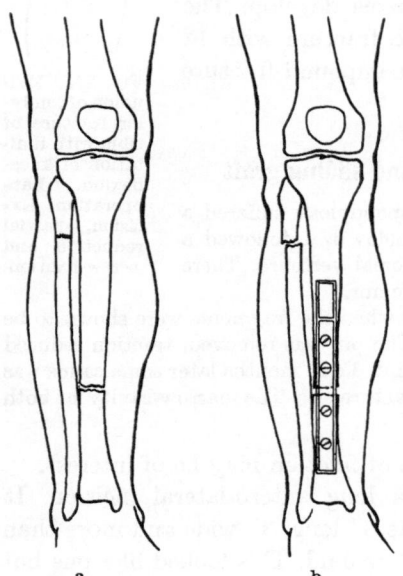

a　　　　　　　　b

Fig. 27a u. b. Pseudarthrosis of tibia. Late operation. Sliding graft fixed with four screws. Fibula refractured

A man aged 26 had a motor-cycle accident causing a fracture-dislocation of T. 11/12 with an incomplete cauda-equina lesion, a rupture of the spleen and a compound comminuted fracture of tibia and fibula, which was infected when he arrived at the Centre. A loose bone splinter sequestrated and had to be removed. After four months' treatment on a splint, the fracture was still fully mobile and the marrow-cavities showed sealing off.

His paralysis had largely recovered and it was doubly important to achieve healing of the fracture without too much shortening. The bone-ends were freshened, a wide sliding graft put across the fracture and fixed with four screws (see BURNS and MICHAELIS 1944). The fibula had to be refractured, since it distracted the fragments of the tibia. Again local spongiosa was packed around the fracture.

Four months later the fracture was firmly healed, with a shortening of 1/3″.

The patient has since been able to walk long distances with sticks and manages a few steps without them. In a very active life the result has been maintained for six years.

Table 28. *Operations in associated fractures. Results*

1. *Early:*	Plating of shaft of humerus	2 Operations	healed, 8 weeks
2. *Late:*	Baldwin's operation of ulna	2 Operations	healed
	Removal of splinters from forearm	1 Operation	healed
	Removal of nerve-compression at wrist	1 Operation	healed
	Open reduction of slipped radial epiphysis	2 Operations	healed
	Open reduction of malunited supracondylar fracture of femur	1 Operation	healed, 2 months
	Open reduction of malunited fracture of tibial condyle	1 Operation	healed, 2 months
	Plating and sliding graft for pseudarthrosis of femur	1 Operation	healed, 6 months
	Sliding graft for pseudarthrosis of tibia	1 Operation	healed, 4 months
		12 Operations	

There was no instance of haemorrhage or infection.

Summary

If indications and techniques of conservative and operative treatment take full account of the special needs of the paraplegic, associated fractures of the long bones heal well, without disabling deformity, and do not interfere with rehabilitation.

2. Late fractures: Indications

The late or secondary fractures of the long bones in paraplegics have been discussed by GUTTMANN (1953), BORS (1955), COMARR, HUTCHINSON and BORS (1959, 1962). A paper on 100 of our cases by GUTTMANN, MELZAK and the author is about to be published.

Here we shall only mention that these fractures occur:

1. With osteoporosis which is due to a combination of protein-loss, anaemia and infection, inactivity and, in patients over 50, presenile changes.
2. In osteomyelitis of the proximal end of femur under pressure-sores.
3. In severely spastic limbs when they are temporarily fixed.
4. In severely toxic children.
5. After severe trauma in the normal bone of incomplete lesions.

Nearly all late fractures of the long bones in paraplegics heal well and rapidly on well-padded, frequently inspected splints, sometimes with a little traction. Blood-transfusion is often needed. We have seen two exceptions belonging to groups 3 and 5 in which operation was indicated.

Case XIV. Fracture of the proximal third of femur with severe spasticity

A corpulent and muscular man aged 50 who was very spastic after a fracture-dislocation of T.7/8/9 vertebrae with an incomplete lesion below T. 6, was admitted one year after his accident with large pressure sores. After we had succeeded in healing them he was, one day, sitting in his wheelchair, gripping his ankle firmly with one hand while trying to put on his shoe with the other. At this moment he had a violent spasm of the hip flexors which broke the femur just below the minor trochanter. During the next few days it became obvious that it was quite impossible to immobilise the proximal fragment, as it was being pulled incessantly with great force in a forward direction. Its sharp point perforated quadriceps and fascia and threatened the skin from within. At the same time there was considerable danger for the femoral vessels.

Nailing might have been possible, but the power of the spasm was such that it might easily have broken either the nail or the wall of the femur. Dr. GUTTMANN decided on an intrathecal alcohol block which produced complete flaccidity. It was now necessary to remove the interposed muscle-mass before good alignment could be achieved. From a long anterolateral incision the fracture was exposed, the sharp points of bone clipped, the quadriceps freed and the bone-ends laid end to end, without removing the remnants of the old haematoma. After closing the incision the leg was immobilised on a wellpadded splint with frequent inspection. Healing occurred within six weeks in good position and with an enormous callus.

The result has been maintained for eleven years.

Case XV. Fracture of the neck of femur in a young man with a very incomplete cauda-equina lesion below L. 4

Fractures of the neck of femur in paraplegics, who are very ill with pressure-sores and urinary infection, are not rare and are always treated conservatively. HOWEVER a young man, aged 24 who, six years after his spinal injury, could walk with sticks, had a severe fall and fractured the neck of femur. We reduced and nailed it with a long, steep nail. The result was complete restoration which has proved to be permanent over the last twelve years.

Small operative measures

In a child of four with multiple fractures and the usual giant callus, there was some reason to suspect a sarcoma. Biopsy confirmed that the fear was unfounded, and the further course corresponded with this.

In a severely toxic man with a flaccid paralysis below T. 2, the spiky fracture-ends of the femur threatened the skin from within. They were blunted from a small incision and the fracture healed in two months.

A girl of 27 suffered an injury to the meniscus of her wrist seven years after a traumatic quadriplegia, incomplete below C. 7. Since she worked as a secretary, pain and swelling made exploration necessary. There has been no swelling since the operation, but pain recurs when she overworks.

Summary

Treatment of late fractures of the long bones in the paraplegic should, with rare exceptions, be conservative. Frequent inspection of the skin, where traction or splints are used, makes considerable demands on the time of the surgeon. But union occurs quickly and with ample callus.

F. Upper limb

Tendon-transfers and arthrodesis of the wrist

In our field there is no more attractive challenge for the surgeon than the paralysis of the long flexors and extensors of the fingers. To be able to give them new power by tendon-transfers or other operations is the ideal task of constructive surgery. Such operations have been carried out successfully by a few surgeons (STREET 1958, NICKEL, PERRY and GARRETT 1963).

Indications

Local restoration of power to carry out isolated functions without loss of general dexterity cannot often be achieved in the quadriplegic, in contrast to patients with flaccid lesions due to poliomyelitis and plexus paralysis. The statement "In a large measure management of upper extremity paralysis is the same, regardless of the cause" (NICKEL, PERRY and GARRETT 1963) is misleading. The loss of sensation and the danger of pressure sores caused by splintage in quadriplegics demand a conservative approach. What they and the sufferers from lower motor neuron lesions have in common, is the need for careful positioning and active and passive movements to wrist and fingers from the first day of neurological involvement onwards. This prevents contractures and limits the indications for operations.

Over the years we are made to understand that, with rare exceptions, even the best-devised operation does not provide a solution which is of real benefit to the patient (ABRAMSON 1953, BORS 1958, STREET 1958, TALBOT 1953 and 1958). Only by observing many quadriplegics for many years do we learn that practice and ingenuity provide a new system of co-ordination between shoulder-elbow-forearm- and wrist movements, and indirect finger-flexion which any operation is bound to disrupt, not merely temporarily. If paralysis is also spastic, operations hardly make sense. Only exceptionally may incomplete lesions with flexor-spasticity make one think of an extensor-transfer to the fingers in order to counteract their flexion.

We have by now treated some four hundred quadriplegics, but only eight operations have been done on six patients. All were free from complications and all achieved at least part of their purpose. However, nearly all have disturbed the new co-ordination so severely, that their value for the patients is doubtful.

I was much impressed by the experience of meeting a young patient from abroad who visited our Centre. She was intelligent, energetic and completely adjusted to her quadriplegia, complete below C. 7. A few years earlier, she had had a series of eight tenodeses and transfers done; these had all been carried out in an exemplary manner.

I observed the actions of this patient without her being aware of it and had to admit that she used almost exclusively the other hand, on which there had been no attempt at surgery. This patient has confirmed my respect for the system of natural adaptation and co-ordination and my scepticism towards operations and complex splints.

Case XVI. Reconstruction of extensor carpi radialis

Another patient, operated on elsewhere, showed in important detail how and when one should *not* operate. A description is called for. In addition, it may be of interest to describe my own operation which was made necessary by the result of the first.

In a car-accident on holiday, the 49-year-old, tall and athletic man broke his cervical spine (C. 4, 5, 6, 7) with a severe but incomplete quadriplegia and concussion. He was flown to this country and treated for the first fourteen months in a well-known orthopaedic centre. His neurological lesion slowly improved.

Eight months after the accident, a surgeon transplanted *ext.* carpi radialis and ulnaris into the superficial and deep flexortendons of the fingers. Healing followed without complication, but the result was crippling. The wrist was fixed in pronounced flexion, the fingers were in clawposition, with maximal hyperextension at the metacarpo-phalangeal joints, and were stiff in flexion at the interphalangeal joints.

When the patient was admitted to us, he had two pressure-sores and a severe adduction-contracture of one hip.

After healing the sores, we first had to do an obturator-neurectomy to enable him to stand and walk. The general anaesthesia given for this operation was used to try and correct the position of the wrist which, however, proved impossible because of contracture and adhesions.

When he started to stand and walk a fortnight later, it became clear that his leg-muscles had regained good power and that he could overcome the spasticity. He could not, however, hold the elbow-crutch. He repeatedly asked us to try and restore useful function to his crippled hand. The other hand and fingers had meanwhile regained a fair degree of active movement and power.

What can we learn from this case?

1. The operation had been done much too early. As long as there is a chance of further improvement in a patient with an incomplete lesion, that is during the first two years, tendon-transfers should not be done except for very unusual reasons.

2. Slight extension of the wrist (10 to 30 degrees) is the optimal position for work with paralysed fingers. The extensors of the wrist alone make this position possible and, therefore, must *never* be transferred on to the flexors.

My plan was to reconstruct the radial extensor-tendon of the wrist and to overcome the contractures by manipulation or, if needed, by operation, so that active extension of the wrist would become possible again.

Operation. At first the old tendon-sutures had to be searched for from the old volar incisions and they were removed. For this first phase I used, as an exception, a tourniquet, which was abandoned as soon as we had found all old sutures. The tendon of extensor carpi ulnaris was left loose. The tendon of extensor carpi radialis was returned to the dorsum of the forearm via its tunnel in which it was fixed by adhesions. From the old dorsal incision it was dissected free and, as expected, proved to be too short.

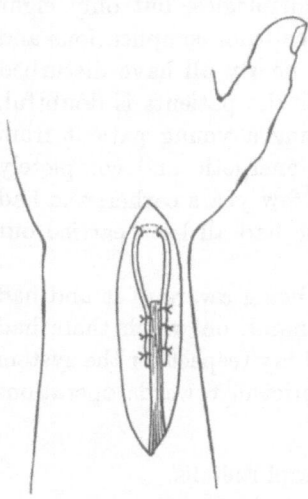

Fig. 28. Reconstruction of tendon of ext. carpi rad. Racket-shaped sling from Palmaris lg. anchored through drill-hole in scaphoid and fixed with wire-sutures at short tendon

It was now possible to manipulate the wrist into full extension. Each finger could be loosened gently. Many adhesions gave way, but postoperative swelling was surprisingly moderate. A four-inch length of tendon of the palmaris longus was fashioned into a racket-shaped sling. This tendon was pulled through a transverse drill-hole in the scaphoid. Both its ends were firmly sutured to the end of the tendon of extensor carpi radialis with the wrist in 30 degrees extension.

A light plaster splint, thickly-padded and removed daily for inspection of pressure-areas, maintained the extension and left the fingers free for active and passive exercises.

Postoperative treatment. Skin sutures were removed after ten days. Two weeks after the operation, gentle active movements of the wrist were started. After a further fortnight the splint was removed for active movements under supervision, but was then reapplied. After altogether six weeks, the splint was applied at night only.

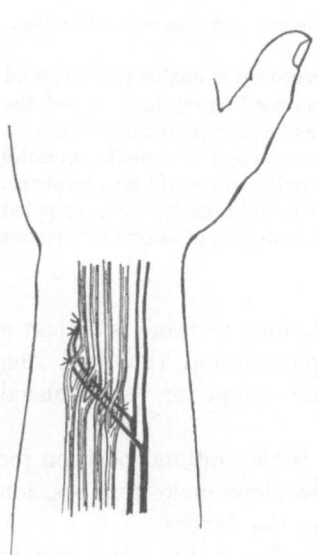

Fig. 29. Tendon-transfer at the wrist

The result was a wrist with full active extension to 30°, active flexion to 10° and active extension and flexion of the fingers with half-normal range and power.

Now, four years later, the result is unchanged. The patient can hold a glass and grip his elbow-crutch well enough to walk for two hours a day.

For over three years, he has been working again in his office as a civil servant.

Tendon-transfers: Operative technique

The other tendon-transfers need not be described in detail (see table 29). In every case the technique consisted in splitting the receptor-tendon, leading the motor-tendon through the slit and fixing it with two wire sutures (gauge 40) in the chosen position of wrist and fingers and at the proper tension. The receptor-tendons were all more or less atrophic.

Case XVII. Arthrodesis of the wrist in a quadriplegic, complete below C. 4/5

In one patient with this very high complete lesion we used a tibial graft for an arthrodesis of his flaccid wrist. He had seen the result of this operation on another patient with poliomyelitis and had only one wish, to be granted a similar firm wrist to enable him to turn over the pages of a book with his knuckles rather than with his wrist. His arthrodesis has done for him what he hoped for during the last four years.

Light well-padded splints may, in the majority of cases, fulfil the same purpose as this operation, but their use demands daily inspection of pressure points. Patients with similarly high lesions are unable to put on or take off these splints by themselves.

If, in exceptional cases only, one undertakes this operation, one must be aware that the small joints of the wrist are very loose in the quadriplegic. The osteoporosis of the small bones does not interfere with prompt healing. However, the

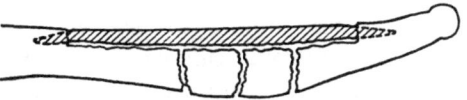

Fig. 30. Arthrodesis of the wrist with tibial graft

graft has to be cut about 1 cm. longer than in the non-paralysed patient. The graft is cut to an arrow-shape at both ends. After thorough preparation of its bed in the radius, the dorsal surfaces of the small bones and the base of the third metacarpal, one should pull fairly hard on the fingers, fit the graft accurately into its bed and then let go of the fingers. Both ends of the graft are thus driven depply into the spongiosa of radius and metacarpus. No further internal fixation is required.

A well-padded volar splint has to be inspected very often. In the absence of bleeding or infection, arthrodesis is complete after three months.

Table 29. *Tendon transfer and Arthrodesis in the upper limb of quadriplegics*

	Neurological Symptomatology and Cause	Age	Operation	Results		Follow-up
				Technical	Functional	
1.	C. 7, incomplete Fracture Dislocation C. 6/7 vertebrae.	20	Fl. carpi. rad. into flex. dig. (bilateral)	Good	Some improvement	9 years
2.	C. 6/7, complete Fracture C. 6 v,	21	Fl. carpi. rad. into fl. dig., ext. carpi. rad. br. into ext. dig.	Good	Little adv.ntage, might need arthrodesis of wrist.	8 years
3.	C 5, incomplete Fracture Dislocation C. 5/6 vertebrae.	26	Ext. carpi. rad. br. into ext. dig.	Good	Doubtful	6 years
4.	C. 4, incomplete Fracture C. 4/5/6 vertebrae	49	Reconstruction of ext. carpi. rad.	Good	Good	4 years
5.	C 5, incomplete Fracture Dislocation C. 6/7 vertebrae.	17	Half of ext. carpi rad. lg. and br. into ext. dig.	Good	Doubtful	4 years
6.	C. 4/5, complete Fracture C 5 v,	19	Arthrodesis of the wrist.	Good	Satisfactory	4 years

Summary

In the last four years among several hundred quadriplegics we have had no occasion to operate on the paralysed wrist or fingers.

Real improvement of function without serious interference with the newly acquired coordination can only rarely be expected.

G. Amputation

There are surgeons (LINDENBERG 1953, CHASE and WHITE 1959) who recommend amputations and exarticulations of the lower limbs for certain paraplegic patients on the grounds that, without their "useless" limbs, they will be more mobile, less dependent and less subject to pressure-sores, contractures and spasticity. They admit that the ability to balance in the sitting position is severely impaired. STREET (1958) also reported on a number of cases.

Dr. GUTTMANN strongly condemns the attitude of surgeons who recommend amputation of the paralysed limbs of paraplegics as a preventive measure in cases of pressure-sores, fractures or spasticity. Indications of this kind are neither scientifically sound nor do they correspond with the principles of modern rehabilitation or, indeed, with humane considerations.

At the Congress of the German Surgical Society at Munich (1959), FELIX again advocated amputation. In his reply Dr. GUTTMANN stated his views and warned against a revival of this method which does nothing but add severe mutilation to paraplegia.

In our material, amputations were carried out on five patients, in two of them bilaterally, for the following four indications:

1. An elderly paraplegic with a cauda-equina lesion also had BUERGER's disease which led to gangrene first in one foot and later in the other. Midthigh amputations prolonged his life for a few years.

2. Two adult patients with low cauda-equina lesions due to myelocele and spina befida had severely stunted and deformed legs below the knees, while the muscles of the thigh, including the quadriceps, were strong. After bilateral below-knee amputation, an 18-year-old girl learned to stand and walk on her prosthesis for the first time in her life and, after a course of bladder-training, now works in a factory (GUTTMANN 1959).

A middle-aged man with a similar lesion was able to walk with a prosthesis after below-knee amputation of one severely deformed leg. He too returned to work.

3. A man whose treatment had been neglected for many years was admitted severely ill with a grotesque deformity of one leg. The hip was ankylosed in extreme abduction and outward rotation while the knee was fixed in an acute flexion-contracture. Furthermore, there was recurrent infective arthritis of the knee-joint due to pressure-sores which endangered his life. Mid-thigh amputation temporarily averted the danger until he died, one year later, of uraemia.

4. A young officer suffered severe open fracture-dislocations of both ankle joints associated with a low spinal injury and an incomplete cauda-equina lesion

below L. 4. While it was possible to obtain healing on one side, severe infection of the joint and osteomyelitis of the lower end of the tibia on the other side made below-knee amputation necessary. With his prosthesis he now walks well with sticks.

All amputations were carried out by another surgeon, (Mr. G. PLATT), except for amputations of five deformed toes which prevented the patients from walking in normal footwear. A further six amputations of toes were carried out by Dr. J. J. WALSH.

We have seen a few instances of amputation in patients who had nothing worse than pressure-sores, and one patient with bilateral exarticulation at the hip who was a pathetic example of the effects of ill-judged surgery and suffered from recurrent pressure-sores on the wasted remnants of his seat.

Literature

The following Monograph is recommended for the study of all aspects of paraplegia:
GUTTMANN, L.: The treatment and rehabilitation of patients with injuries of the spinal cord. Vol. Surgery, Medical History of the 2nd World War, pp. 422—516. H. M. Stationary Office 1953.

References of individual papers

ABRAMSON, A. S.: J. Bone Jt Surg. 30-A, 932 (1948)
— Proc. clin. Parapl. Conf. (1953); (1955).
— Arch. phys. Med. 43, 147 (1961).
— Changing concepts in the management of spasticity; in: J. D. FRENCH and R. W. PORTER, eds.: Basic research in paraplegia, pp. 205—227. Springfield (Ill.): Thomas 1962.
— and DELAGE: Res. Quart. 31, 365 (1960).
— and Hirschberg: Bull Hosp. Jt Dis. (N.Y.) 164—172 (1952)
— and KAMBERG: J. Bone Jt Surg. 31-A, 275 (1949)
ARMSTRONG-RESSY, C. T., A. A. WEISS, and A. EBEL: Proc. Clin. Parapl. Conf. (1957).
— — — N.-Y. St. J. Med. 59, 2548 (1959).
BÉNASSY, J.: Rev. Rhum. 24, 457 (1957).
— J. R. BOISSIER, D. PATTE, and J. C. DIVERRES: Presse med. 811—814 (1960).
— J. C. DIVERRES, D. PATTE, and J. DENIS: Ann. Med. Phys. 3, 4 (1960).
— and A. MEZABRAUD: Rev. Rhum. 234—240 (1961).
— and J. C. DIVERRES: Rev. Chir. orthop. 49, 95—116 (1963).
BERNSON, J.: Proc. clin. Parapl. Conf. 72 (1956).
BIESALSKI, K., and L. MAYER: Die physiologische Sehnenverpflanzung. Berlin: Springer 1916.
BORS, E.: Proc. clin. Parapl. Conf. 46 (1955); (1958).
— Proc. clin. Spinal Cord Inj. Conf. (1959); (1960).
BROWN, A. S.: Lancet 1958/II, 975—978.
BURKE, J.: Wien. klin. Wschr. 72, 749—750 (1960).
BURNS, B. H., and L. S. MICHAELIS: Lancet 1944/I, 337.
CEILLIER, A.: Para-ostéo-arthropathies des paraplégiques par lésions de la moelle épinière et de la queue de cheval. Thèse 296 (1920)
CHASE, R. A., and W. L. WHITE: Plast. reconstr. Surg. 24, 445 (1959).
COMARR, A. E.: Proc. clin. Parapl. Conf. (1958).
— Proc. Clin. Spinal Cord Inj. Conf. (Surg. f. Spasticity) (1960).
— Amer. J. Surg. 103, 732 (1962).
— R. H. HUTCHINSON and E. BORS: Proc. Clin. Spinal Cord Inj. Conf. (Statistics of fractures) 53 (1959).

DAMANSKI, M.: J. Bone Jt Surg. 43, 286 (1961).
DÉJÉRINE, C. A.: Rev. neurol. 25, 159, 207, 348 (1918).
— Ann. Med. 5, 497 (1919).
— Rev. neurol. 26, 399 (1900).
DOGLIOTTI, A. M.: Proposta di un nuovo metodo di cura delle algie periferiche. Minerva med.
    1, 636 (1931).
EBEL, A.: Proc. clin. Parapl. Conf. (1956).
EICHENHOLTZ, S. N.: Management of long-bone fractures in paraplegic patients. J. Bone Jt
    Surg. 45-A, 299 (1963).
EICHHORST, H.: Virchows Arch. path. Anat. 139, 193 (1895).
FINKELMANN, T.: Proc. clin. Parapl. Conf. (1956).
FINKLE, J. R.: Proc. clin. Parapl. Conf. (1956); (1960).
FOWLER, A. W.: 7th World Congr. Soc. Welf. of Cripples, Report p. 429, 1957.
FREEHAFER, A. A., R. LOWRY, and TH. F. LINKE: Proc. clin. Spinal Cord Inj. Conf. (1961).
GINGRAS, G., J. M. MCINTYRE, and M. MONGEAU: Orthopedic surgery in the rehabilitation
    of paraplegics. Treat. Serv. Bull. Ottowa 7, 438 (1952).
GUTTMANN, L.: J. Bone Jt Surg. 31-B, 389 (1949).
— Monograph, see above (1953).
— Dtsch. Z. Nervenheilk 175, 173—190 (1956)
— Die Rehabilitation von Querschnittsgelähmten des Rückenmarks. Dtsch. med. J. 7, 326
    (1956).
— Proc. Roy. Soc. Med. 50, 742 (1959).
— Langenbecks Arch. klin. Chir. 298, 187 (1961).
— and P. MEDAWAR: J. Neurol. Psychiat. 5, 13 (1942).
HALL, R. H.: Proc. clin. Parapl. Conf. (1953).
HARDY, A. G.: Proc. Roy. Soc. Med. 52, 802 (1959).
— and J. W. DICKSON: Pathological ossification in traumatic paraplegia. J. Bone Jt Surg.
    45-B, 76 (1963).
HASS, J.: Zbl. Chir. 43, 2702 (1925).
— Langenbecks Arch. klin. Chir. 60, 693 (1930).
— J. Bone Jt Surg. 26, 297 (1944).
KELLY, R. E., and P. GAUTHIER-SMITH: Lancet 1959/II, 1102.
KUETTNER, H.: Berl. klin. Wschr. 45, 654 (1908).
LINDENBERG, W.: Nervenarzt 24, 127 (1953).
LODGE, T.: Acta radiol. (Stockh.) 435 (1957).
MACEWEN, G. D., and R. G. UNDERDAL: Heterotopic ossification in paraplegia. Case report.
    Delaware med. J. 34, 113 (1962).
MAHER, R. M.: Lancet 1955/I, 18.
MASSE, P.: Rev. Chir. (Paris) 34 (1958).
— Mém. Acad. Chir. 977 (1958).
MERLE D'AUBIGNÉ, H., et J. BÉNASSY: in „Chir. Orth. des Paralysies". Paris: Masson 1958.
MICHAELIS, L. S.: Proc. Roy. Soc. Med. 47 (1954); 52 (1959).
MILLËR, L. F.: Proc. clin. Parapl. Conf. 19 (1956).
— and C. J. O'NEILL: J. Bone Jt Surg. 31-A, 283 (1949).
NATHAN, P. W., and T. G. SCOTT: Lancet 1958/I, 76; 1959/II, 1099.
NICKEL, V. L., J. PERRY, and A. L. GARRETT: J. Bone Jt Surg. 45-A, 933—952 (1963).
NISSEN-LIE, H. S.: J. Oslo Cy Hosp. 3, 186 (1953).
POURPRE, H.: Neuro-Chirurgie 6, 229 (1960).
SCHNEIDER, M., and A. D. KRUG: J. Bone Jt Surg. 42-A, 1165 (1960).
SELIG, R.: Langenbecks Arch. klin. Chir. 103, 994 (1914).
STAMM, T. T.: Proc. Roy. Soc. Med. 35, 221 (1942).
STEHMANN, M.: Acta orthop. belg. 3, 207 (1959).
ŠTĚPÁNEK, V., and P. ŠTĚPÁNEK: Changes in the bones and joints of paraplegics. Radiol. clin.
    (Basel) 29, 28 (1960).
STREET, D. M.: Proc. clin. Parapl. Conf. 9 (1958).
TALBOT, H. S.: Proc. clin. Parapl. Conf. 30 (1953); (1958).

Index

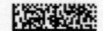